Mad

'In these urgent times, activists are often seeking guidance on radical approaches to mental health. *Mad World* offers a welcome and refreshing guide to a progressive politics of mental health – an indispensable resource for activists today.'

—Hel Spandler, Editor, *Asylum: The Radical Mental Health Magazine*

'Wow! An honest, urgent and lovingly researched invitation to rethink our assumptions about madness. *Mad World* is an invaluable toolkit, not just for dismantling oppressive health structures, but for building the systems of care we desperately need. This book is a gift and that gift is hope.'

—Aisha Mirza, founder of Misery mental health collective

'Really brilliant ... this is by far the best introduction to mad politics I've ever read.'

—Robert Chapman, Senior Lecturer in Education, Sheffield Hallam University

'An urgent introduction to a new radical politics of mental health which embraces the messy, unruly nature of our collective vulnerability and interdependence. Frazer-Carroll exposes the underlying truth that capitalism is fundamentally incompatible with our wellbeing. *Mad World* teaches us how to transform the ways we understand madness, illness, and disability to build a better world.'

—Beatrice Adler-Bolton, co-author of *Health Communism*

Outspoken by Pluto
Series Editor: Neda Tehrani

Platforming underrepresented voices; intervening in important political issues; revealing powerful histories and giving voice to our experiences; Outspoken by Pluto is a book series unlike any other. Unravelling debates on feminism and class, work and borders, unions and climate justice, this series has the answers to the questions you're asking. These are books that dissent.

Also available:

Mad World
The Politics of Mental Health

Micha Frazer-Carroll

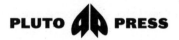
PLUTO PRESS

First published 2023 by Pluto Press
New Wing, Somerset House, Strand, London WC2R 1LA
and Pluto Press, Inc.
1930 Village Center Circle, 3-834, Las Vegas, NV 89134

www.plutobooks.com

British Library Cataloguing in Publication Data
A catalogue record for this book is available from the British Library

ISBN   978 0 7453 4671 7   Paperback
ISBN   978 0 7453 4674 8   PDF
ISBN   978 0 7453 4672 4   EPUB
ISBN   978 0 7453 4849 0   Audio

This book is printed on paper suitable for recycling and made from
fully managed and sustained forest sources. Logging, pulping and
manufacturing processes are expected to conform to the environmen-
tal standards of the country of origin.

Typeset by Stanford DTP Services, Northampton, England

Simultaneously printed in the United Kingdom and United States of
America

Contents

Acknowledgements

The birth of this book has made me deeply anxious. It has been maddening in many ways – the writing process sent me around in circles, saw me retreat inside my home and isolate myself from others, kept me up at night in a panic. However, books are collectively made. A sprawling community of people held me through this experience, also contributing their time and perspectives to the book. Despite my name on the spine, this book would not have been possible without those who supported both my writing process and/or my emotional process: Mum, Dad, Pascale Frazer-Carroll, Nathan Frazer-Carroll, Hassanali Pesaran, Lola Olufemi, Georgia Elander, Florence Oulds, Robert Chapman, Amelia Horgan, Ella Asheri, Alice Markham, Doris Cozma, Waithera Sebatindira, Lauren Corelli, Leah Cowan, Hel Spandler, Emily Reynolds, Miriam Gauntlett, Akanksha Mehta, Maya Wolfe-Robinson, Esther Kaner, Martha Krish, Adam Almeida, Campaign for Psych Abolition (CPA) and David Jones. A special thank you to Edi, my first reader, who kept me afloat throughout this process. I'd also like to extend gratitude to the Wellcome Collection, whose archivists assisted my work. Of course, this book would not have been possible without my editor, Neda Tehrani, who has supported and been patient with me since our first conversation in 2019. It would be impossible for this book to represent the united views of each of these people and all the names quoted inside it. There is too much breadth of experience and contestation. I have drawn on many people's ideas and what is compiled here is an offering, which I hope will be a jumping off point for the next person. All errors are my own.

Introduction

One morning, in the summer of 2016, my mind split in half. As I opened my eyes to bring the day into focus, the same way I had done every single day of my life so far, I couldn't quite make things sharp enough. It was as if I hadn't fully awoken to 'reality', but was stuck in some liminal purgatory between the dreaming and waking worlds. Everything looked as if it was taking place on a television screen – myself, an audience member watching my own life play out from afar. As the days, weeks and months dragged on, I couldn't shake this dizzy, detached and anxious feeling, and began to spiral into panic attacks multiple times a day. I found myself in a living nightmare, feeling not-quite-dead but not alive either, resigned to the idea that I would either have to relinquish life or accept this new waking death. This experience, which lifted after a number of months, was in retrospect one of the most destabilising yet significant periods of my life. It was a time in which I went mad.

There is a clinical name for what I was experiencing: 'depersonalisation disorder', a state of 'dissociation' that is linked to extreme anxiety levels. People who experience depersonalisation for a long period, like I did, often express relief upon this realisation that they have not 'gone mad'. But to me, it was undoubtedly madness; I could feel it in my mind and I could see it in the way that people looked at me when I tried to explain my predicament. Lacking a strong community around me, and conscious of my 'unpalatable' form of distress, I intuitively swallowed my madness. I only dared to utter it in interactions with various professionals, while treading precariously around the scripted questions that determine whether a person will be sectioned. For so many others like myself, madness and mental distress is an overwhelmingly isolating endeavour under our current conditions. It can cut us off from our communities, make us feel trapped, take over our lives, and see us further secluded within the system – both physically and metaphorically. It can pile on shame, disgust and trauma, turning our days into a struggle to simply stay alive. How, then, do we take such alienating and debilitating experiences and turn them outwards to politicise them?

This is the central concern that this book attempts to tackle. In recent decades, we have seen an explosion of liberal 'mental health awareness' campaigns, demanding that we 'speak out' and 'break the stigma' around mental health. A slew of memoirs and confessional mental health writing has also followed, dissecting the personal dimensions of distress and providing many of us with narratives that we can 'relate' to. Others have begun to interrogate the link between oppression and mental health – for example, the relationship between race, gender and distress. Most of these discussions, however, are yet to make political, historical and economic analyses that are truly radical and grasp problems at the root. While currents in mental health conversations may have shifted and swirled about on the surface, the deep, murky water beneath largely remains the same. We are yet to sufficiently grapple with questions like: how does my experience link to yours? What shared structures and material conditions dictate how we all understand and experience what we call madness or mental illness? What even is madness/mental illness, and should we take these constructs at face value?

This book mobilises anti-capitalist, 'mad', disability justice and anti-racist thinking in particular to carve out a radical political approach to mental health. It names the capitalist economic system, specifically, as a significant producer of suffering in contemporary life. Capitalism, a system character-ised by private ownership, wage labour, competition and the pursuit of profit, harms each and every one of us. It separates us – workers – from our work; forces us to choose between inhumane working conditions or death; pushes people into dangerous living conditions and houselessness; destroys our environment; sanctions and normalises all kinds of death; forces the unemployed into murderous benefits systems and social institutions; and allows a limited few to accumulate more wealth than they could ever need. Around 10% of the world lives in extreme poverty.[1] These conditions are largely inflicted on women, young people, children and people living in the 'Global South'.[2] One hundred million people are estimated to be homeless worldwide, and as many as 1.6 billion lack adequate housing.[3] More than 60% of workers worldwide are in temporary, part-time or short-term jobs in which wages are falling.[4] Neoliberal austerity has seen healthcare, youth centres, housing budgets and benefits slashed, depriving us from access to bodily autonomy, community, safety, dignity and joy. This is the context in which depression has become the leading global cause of disability.[5] Under these conditions, life is not only unfulfilling for many, but also unliveable.

---

1   https://worldbank.org/en/topic/poverty/overview (last accessed January 2023).

2   https://worldvision.org/sponsorship-news-stories/global-poverty-facts (last ac-cessed January 2023).

3   https://homelessworldcup.org/homelessness-statistics (last accessed January 2023).

4   https://www.solidaritycenter.org/ilo-precarious-work-rises-incomes-fall-around-the-world/ (last accessed January 2023)

5   https://who.int/news-room/fact-sheets/detail/depression (last accessed January 2023).

On a psychological and interpersonal level, capitalism affects all of us. It infiltrates and corrupts how we fundamentally think about one another. The insidious logics of extraction, exploitation, scarcity and competition impact on how we talk, befriend, date and otherwise interact with each other. Capitalism birthed even the most commonplace social structures in which we distribute care, abuse and resources. It is no coincidence that the Western capitalist nuclear family unit is the institution that psychoanalysts have long located at the epicentre of our neuroses. Intimate relationships and marriages – another normalised economic unit – often produce trauma. In this sense, and many others, capitalism fractures community, laying the foundations for isolation and abuse. Its allied systems, for example, white supremacy and ableism, also trap and harm us on a psychic level. It is only years following my experience of depersonalisation that I can look back and see that it was connected to intergenerational trauma, racism, ableism, abuse, work, and my lack of a caring community. The Diagnostic and Statistical Manual of Mental Disorders (DSM), psychiatry's age-old manual of 'mental disorders' says of depersonalisation: 'The individual may feel detached from his or her entire being (e.g., "I am no one," "I have no self").'[6] I have come to believe that my own identity collapse was a response to my untenable personal and political conditions at the time. My consciousness 'split off' as some form of escape.

The bodyworker Lisa Fannen describes capitalism itself as a dissociative state: 'Many of us were made to sit still for long periods of time at school, engaging predominantly with our rational "minds", when we might have had strong impulses

---

6 American Psychiatric Association, *Diagnostic and Statistical Manual of Mental Disorders*, fifth edition, 2013.

to run/move/dream.'[7] As Fannen observes, we all have to find internal survival mechanisms to escape our harmful conditions from an early age. Few of us know how it feels to genuinely be free, to be self-directed, to live without fear of punishment or violence, and to really flourish. We must all 'dissociate' to some extent – smiling for our employers and crying about it in therapy; tolerating daily microaggressions and venting about it within our communities; exhaling when we arrive home and feel able to finally remove our mask. Few of us can safely and fully exist in this world, and the mental toll catches up with us.

This book does not, however, only chart how oppressive systems harm our mental health. It also aims to push us further, to interrogate how 'mental health' is constructed in itself. A truly political approach cannot only look at *causes* of what we call madness or mental illness. It must also be 'constructivist' – interrogating the very concepts of madness and mental illness themselves, prizing them apart, questioning their function. We have no shortage of conflicting messages dictating what mental illness is: it is discussed as a chemical imbalance in the brain, as something that doesn't exist, as a product of capitalism alone, as akin to a broken leg, as a social construct, as something that is physical and real. To address these contradictions, we must ask: Where did the concepts of madness and mental illness come from? Who do they serve? In a different world, how might these categories be transformed? Looking at mental illness as a 'social construct' does not mean that these experiences are not 'real' but rather that they do not constitute a fixed or objective category across time and space. Like race, like gender, like all illness and other forms of deviance from the norm,[8] the concepts

---

7   L. Fannen, *Warp And Weft: Psycho-Emotional Health, Politics And Experiences*, (N.P.: Active Distribution, 2021).

8   P. Sedgwick, *PsychoPolitics* (London: Pluto Press, 1982, 2022).

of madness and mental illness have been moulded in a particular social, political and economic context, and would look different in a liberated future.

Taking a radical approach to mental health also means drawing on a long history of political agitation in this area. Throughout the mid-late twentieth century, there was a groundswell of activism and contestation around mental health – in the form of the 'anti-psychiatry' and 'psychiatric survivor' movements, which shared some overlap with other liberation movements of the time. Both movements challenged psychiatry (the dominant medical approach to mental health), arguing that suffering should be seen as a social and political concern rather than an individual one. They also resisted psychiatric power and control, which had allowed for the mass incarceration of mad or mentally ill people in giant 'insane asylums' or 'mental hospitals'. From a present-day perspective, it is curious that the histories of these political movements have been erased, while the movements have left little imprint on the ways that mental health is approached and understood today. In the current climate, we still largely discuss mental health in terms of individual identity (something we *are*) and property ownership (something we *have*) – rather than as a form of collective oppression (something that is done to us). Even in political spaces that are suspicious of state authority, deference to psychiatric ideas is very much the norm. We are scared to touch mental health, usually out of fear of getting the 'science' wrong. I have noticed some of the most vocal and political people I know confess that they lack 'expertise' or 'authority' on mental health, despite the fact that suffering surrounds us in our communities.

This fear and avoidance, however, reinforces madness and mental illness as a private matter that we must outsource to other institutions. This is the capitalist approach to mental health in disguise; the force that pushed people out of communities and into asylums, disappearing them from public view. Many commonplace utterances around mental health are also distinctly neoliberal – for example, it is standard and even sometimes considered humorous to urge people to 'get therapy' or even to 'take their meds' when they are understood to be causing harm or disruption. This echoes the gradual shift in mental health provision towards private for-profit entities over the last half a century. When we frame mental health in such a way, we bolster the idea that it is each person's individual responsibility to stay well by seeking out therapists, psychiatrists, psychologists, doctors, self-help books, crisis lines and more recently apps and self-care gurus, many of which are becoming increasingly ubiquitous and profitable in the neoliberal era. While these things may help many survive or conform to the construct of 'mental health', they will never address the root causes of suffering or harm. They also cannot provide us with the tools to transform the world that drives so many of us mad.

While writing this book, I never found the perfect language to describe its subject matter. At the time of writing, 'mental health problems' is perhaps the dominant term – simultaneously shirking and embracing the language of 'illness'. Some prefer 'mental illness', and feel that it accurately describes their experiences. In the pages that follow, we will also look at movements that deplored the concept of mental illness, arguing that it is either oppressive or unscientific. This book offers autonomy to the reader in making sense of these contentions. It shows that, while the state currently favours 'illness' as an explanation for some forms of suffering and nonconformity, it is not the only way of thinking about these experiences. Simultaneously, it acknowledges that illness can be a site of political analysis and solidarity. I want to hold space for lots of different conceptualisations and possibilities. I also want to honour the different language used to describe these experiences across time – for example, for much of history, the term 'madness' had a specific and historically significant meaning. To reflect these competing demands, and for the purposes of brevity, I choose to refer to 'Madness/Mental Illness' throughout this book. I understand that both of these terms carry loaded and personal connotations for many of us, and that their implications will change across time. From here onwards, I also choose to capitalise the first letter of these words – to ensure we never lose sight of the fact that these are highly political and constructed categories, which have been birthed and named by people. In instances where I utilise diagnostic terminology, for example, 'depression' or 'bipolar', I also carry an awareness that these categories are constructed and contested, and try, where possible, to do justice to this. Ultimately, I ask that we sit with the imperfect and ever-changing nature of language, and also take stock of what it tells us about this highly political subject.

Many of the arguments in the pages that follow are guided by my commitment to the disability justice movement, a movement pioneered by disabled people of colour, which takes a radical and intersectional approach to the liberation of disabled people.[9] Some of the more unconventional arguments I make – which simultaneously resist psychiatric control, but also challenge historical 'anti-psychiatry' movements – are unique precisely because they are grounded in disability justice. This approach also informs my language choices. For example, there is a tendency in mental health discourses to cleave a hard line between mental and physical, and mind from body. In line

---

9   See '10 Principles of Disability Justice' by Sins Invalid for a more detailed account: https://sinsinvalid.org/blog/10-principles-of-disability-justice (last accessed January 2023).

with other disabled thinkers, I want to contest Western mind-body dualism; and so throughout this book, I generally refer to complete 'bodyminds'.

Each sentence contained within the following pages relates to a set of concerns that may cease to exist in a world that was transformed. This book grapples with issues like the incarceration and punishment of Mad/Mentally Ill people; the emergence of these approaches under the capitalist system; the push to understand Madness/Mental Illness in one, restricted way; the maddening nature of racism, transphobia and wage labour; and the pathologisation of marginalised people. All of these issues are tied to what are sometimes called the psychiatric and medical industrial complexes – systems that emerged under capitalism to largely serve capitalist ends. In a different world, our conditions could be transformed beyond recognition, and so it follows that our approaches to mental health would also be unrecognisable. We could be in control of our own labour, our own healthcare, our own healing, we could choose how we name ourselves rather than having labels enforced on us. We could ensure that everyone had the resources, infrastructure and support to live in the community. Resources could be reallocated in such a way that health would flood out of closed spaces and into everyday life. Our living and labouring conditions could lead far fewer people to suffering and sickness in the first place. Our conception of mental health could be transformed too.

This book is an offering, not a comprehensive instruction manual. Throughout the writing process, I have grappled with its limits as a commodity that demands I, the *writer*, speak to you, the *reader*. I want to resist this relationship in the same way that I resist the concepts of knowledgeable expert versus ignorant layperson or doctor versus patient. While this is not a personal piece of writing, my experiences weave their way throughout this linear form, to challenge the role of omniscient writer and locate the subjective position that I speak from. This book has also led me to grapple with the bounds of the current mental health conversation, and therefore all that will be left unsaid in this concise exploration. This is only exacerbated by my position as someone writing from a limited British Global North perspective. Regardless, I hope that this book will be a jumping off point. I offer it with humility. There will be holes in it,[10] contradictions, cycles and repetitions, things that in the future are discovered to be inaccurate, incomplete, blinkered or a product of their time. This reflects the spirit of Madness, but that is okay, because this project demands a sort of Mad thinking. After all, what is the utility of 'sanity' or 'rationality', in a world in which 'sanity' means the death of oppressed people and the planet,[11] and 'rationality' means the logic of the market? In this climate, it is Madness that will help us burst beyond the 'rational' confines of the asylum, of the prison, of capitalism and individualism. As the world drives us increasingly Mad, it is crucial that we take Mad knowledge seriously, and acknowledge its imaginative potential. This journey began when I woke up in a dissociative dream. I believe various forms of dissociation, dreaming and escape from this world are the only way to transform it.

---

10 https://gutsmagazine.ca/in/ (last accessed January 2023).

11 I borrow this suggestion from the psychiatric survivor David Oaks: https://davidwoaks.com/july-mad-pride-and-disability-pride-month (last accessed January 2023).

Chapter 1

Asylums

How do we learn to not see what we see, or to not know what we know? – Clair Wills

One day, while I was walking outside Liverpool Street Station in London, I noticed a blue, rectangular tile on a white strip of wall, sandwiched between an events venue and a wine bar. Its block capitals read: 'SITE OF THE FIRST BETHLEHEM HOSPITAL, 1247–1676'. Growing up, my only route into central London had been via a train to Liverpool Street, and so I had unknowingly walked past this plaque for years, never really noticing it. But, while going for a McDonald's as I waited for my train, or running to catch the last departure home, I never knew that I was standing in Bethlem (or 'Bedlam'), the world's first institution for the Mad. I had also therefore never given a thought to the people who had been locked up on the very ground I was walking on. Standing face to face with this plaque, I felt confronted by a history that few of us really know, despite all our talk of the importance of mental health today.

My ignorance, all of our ignorance, about this history, is also reflected in the interests of historians. For lots of the twentieth century, the history of mental health was mainly written in academic forums by psychiatrists – and they almost exclusively wrote it in a way that was tainted by their current beliefs: a slow forward march from a dark and brutal past to a kind, enlightened present.[1] It wasn't until 1961, when the philosopher Michel Foucault published *Madness and Civilisation*, in the early days of a growing movement against psychiatry, that the tides began to turn in the popular imagination. As part of his interrogation, Foucault didn't take Madness as a given, pointing out that the saints, holy fools and court jesters of one era seemed to be viewed as the 'lunatics' of the next. He argued that Madness wasn't an 'objective' entity, it was something unstable that changed across time. Other thinkers also started to reflect on and publish popular books on the treatment of Mad people across history, and the origins of the asylum system, which was still very much ongoing.

Shortly after this flurry of interest in Madness and asylums in the 1960s and 70s, the asylums that were peppered across each one of Britain's counties began to be dismantled by the state. Since this period, dubbed 'deinstitutionalisation', these political discussions about asylums have largely vanished once again from the collective consciousness. Today, depictions of asylums in the horror genre make a mockery of institutionalisation, presenting asylums as eerie gothic settings, which are often completely empty of human residents. Comedies and popular cartoons feature jokes about straitjackets, lobotomies and padded cells. In one episode of *The Simpsons*, Homer is even carted off to the 'New Bedlam Insane Asylum'. This empathy gap floods out into the 'real world' too – one of the popular student nightclubs at my university advertised a Halloween event with the theme 'The Asylum'.[2]

---

1   R. Porter, 'Madness and society in England: the historiography reconsidered', *Studies in History*, 3:2, (1987), pp. 275–90.

2   https://thetab.com/2015/09/09/clueless-cambridge-society-organises-asylum-night-in-the-middle-of-refugee-crisis-52896 (last accessed January 2023).

We should interrogate our numbness to the concept of the asylum, and the way we often think about it as a sort of fictional terror or a relic of the past. I start this book with the history of asylums because, while it is easy to forget them, they are the foundation on which we have built our current understanding and treatment of mental health.[3] We are walking near asylum grounds every day, and walking among the legacy of the asylum too.

'Bedlam'

Bethlem, the first institution to house the 'insane', was originally established to care for 'sick paupers', but by the fifteenth century, it had begun to specialise in Madness. There is a lot of evidence to suggest that the people housed at Bethlem were subjected to extremely brutal treatment. Some accounts report restraint, whipping and people being made to sleep on beds of straw. In 1403, one charity commissioners report stated that there were four pairs of manacles (shackles), eleven chains, six locks and two pairs of stocks (a type of wooden board placed around the ankles and wrists) at the institution.[4] But crucially, there were only six insane residents – asylums were not a large part of medieval society.

Even by the seventeenth century, institutionalisation was exceptionally rare, with resident numbers creeping up to 21 in a country with a population of a few million.[5] Most Mad people – a broad and poorly defined category that might include ailments

---

3   I take a British focus, in particular, because Britain is where the asylum began, later to be exported across the world.

4   J. Andrews, A. Briggs, R. Porter, P. Tucker and K. Waddington, *The History of Bethlem* (Abingdon: Routledge, 1998).

5   E. F. Torrey, 'The Rise of Cats and Madness: II. The Seventeenth and Eighteenth Centuries', *Parasites, Pussycats and Psychosis* (Cham: Springer, 2022).

such as 'bad marriages', 'hatred of spouse', 'mopishness', 'possession by spirits', 'witchcraft', visions or 'melancholy'[6] – were cared for by their families or their broader communities. To understand this, we need to understand the context of England before capitalism. In a feudal society, in which work generally consisted of agriculture or small-scale industry, work was slower, and people had a degree of control over their working conditions. Therefore Mad people and other disabled people were often able to contribute to the production process to some degree or another.[7]

In the latter half of the seventeenth century, population growth, economic change and the rapid expansion of the capital into neighbouring villages meant that many families found themselves unable to host their Mad relatives.[8] Bethlem became overrun with applications, and needed to expand to accommodate the growing numbers of Mad people, whose families often admitted them to be institutionalised. Since Bethlem had such low capacity, a number of private 'madhouses' began to spring up to plug the gap,[9] and in the latter half of the century, a renowned architect named Robert Hooke was commissioned to design a new, much larger Bethlem, which would accommodate 136 patients near Moorgate, in the City of London.

The second incarnation of Bethlem was a giant, palace-like building in the heart of London, designed in an opulent baroque

---

6   L. Kassell, M. Hawkins, R. Ralley, J. Young, J. Edge, J. Yvonne Martin-Portugues and N. Kaoukji (eds), *The Casebooks of Simon Forman and Richard Napier, 1596–1634: A Digital Edition*, https://casebooks.lib.cam.ac.uk.

7   M. Oliver, 'The Politics of Disablement — New Social Movements', *The Politics of Disablement: Critical Texts in Social Work and the Welfare State* (Palgrave: London, 1990).

8   P. Chambers, *Bedlam: London's Hospital for the Mad* (Hersham: Ian Allan Publishing, 2009).

9   R. Porter, 'Madness and society in England: the historiography reconsidered', *Studies in History*, 3:2, (1987), pp. 275–90.

style, with the façade of the building inspired by Louis XIV's Tuileries Palace in Paris. The idea of a palace for Mad people unsurprisingly attracted some ridicule upon the building's rapid completion and opening in 1676.[10] Some mockingly compared it to the Palace of Versailles, questioning how appropriate its design was for its purpose.[11] But, on the contrary, the state was setting out its ideological vision for Madness, and the way that it would relate to Mad people.

We should remember that the new Bethlem didn't only serve the function of warehousing the Mad – it also had an image to keep up with the general public. As was the case on the old site, the building in Moorgate would also serve as a visitor attraction, and would benefit from spectators' donations.[12] While lots of people have framed this visitation as a grotesque sort of 'museum of the Mad',[13] where cruel members of the general public would pay to gawk at Mad people like zoo animals, what was taking place was more insidious than that. Bethlem's public image – its system of visitation, astonishing architecture and location in the heart of London – all helped create the necessary myths to legitimise and sustain the brutal emerging system. For example, the asylum's public visibility was a reminder of the grave consequences of non-conformity to the emerging societal order.[14,15] Simultaneously, Bethlem's costly architecture and central

---

10   R. Mindham, 'Robert Hooke's Bethlem Hospital of 1676: An architectural wonder—psychiatry in pictures', *British Journal of Psychiatry*, 218:4, (2021), p. 181.

11   Ibid.

12   J. Andrews, A. Briggs, R. Porter, P. Tucker, K. Waddington, *The History of Bethlem* (Abingdon: Routledge, 1998).

13   A. Scull, *The Most Solitary of Afflictions: Madness and Society in Britain, 1700–1900* (New Haven: Yale University Press, 1993).

14   J. Andrews, *Bedlam Revisited: A History of Bethlem Hospital 1634–1770* (Thesis, University of London, 1991).

15   A. Scull, 'Madness and Segregative Control: The Rise of the Insane Asylum', *Social Problems*, 24:3, (1977), 337–51.

location helped bolster the idea that 'care' for the Mad was a noble mission, of primary importance to society. The historian Jonathan Andrews also argues that by visiting Bethlem, people may have felt that they were engaging in a charitable endeavour, by witnessing the plight of the Mad and then making a donation to the institution (which was encouraged).[16]

While it is easy to say that none of this continues today, as Andrews suggests, we can try to connect the dots between then and now. Bethlem, which is still a psychiatric institution that stands in South London, may no longer quite be the 'museum of the Mad' that it was then. But would you believe that it still remains open to day trippers, who can walk its grand grounds and attend its exhibit called the 'Museum of the Mind'? That the museum has its own TripAdvisor page? While visitors may not go to look at living patients, in the museum, they can learn about the unthinkable historical conditions of the very same asylum residents that spectators once went to visit. They can reflect on the appearance of progress across the centuries, while present-day patients are detained in the next building.

Into the eighteenth century, people continued to be put through torturous treatments within the walls of the 'palace' for the Mad. 'Humoral' treatments for Madness were rife; the idea was that, by expelling certain humours (blood, black bile, yellow bile and phlegm) from the body, they could balance people's minds. This usually meant a gruelling itinerary of bleeding, vomiting and laxatives, sometimes accompanied by other types of purging, like the burning and the blistering of the skin.[17] Other treatments included 'rotational therapy', which involved suspending a patient from the ceiling and spinning them at up

---

16 Andrews, *Bedlam Revisited*.

17 P. Chambers, *Bedlam: London's Hospital for the Mad* (Hersham: Ian Allan Publishing, 2009).

to 100 rotations per minute, for hours at a time, sometimes also inducing vomiting.[18] Some people within the asylum remained chained to walls. The asylum was also kept icily cold, due to the supposed sedative effects of cool temperatures. The medical rationale then was similar to what it is now: that treatment, no matter how painful or non-consensual, is justified as long as it stands a chance of producing the outcome of 'cure'.

However, the inhumane conditions at Bethlem, and the extremely painful and invasive physical treatments at the hospital, were not without criticism during this period. One leading progressive 'Mad doctor', William Battie, published a famous work called *A Treatise on Madness* in 1758, in which he mostly critiqued the treatment of incarcerated Bedlamites. The ability for people to visit and see these conditions for themselves also added fuel to this fire, and a growing asylum reform movement began to pick up steam. In 1814, the Quaker Edward Wakefield visited Bethlem, and famously discovered a patient called James Norris,[19] who had allegedly been shackled to his bed at Bethlem for 14 years. The case was widely reported in the press – and soon after, a parliamentary select committee was set up to address the inhumane conditions of people living in public asylums and private madhouses.

The discrepancy between Bethlem's proud exterior, and the true dilapidation of its interior, was also beginning to take hold of the building itself. The asylum, which had once been an awe-inspiring, highly visible building, whose name had become synonymous with chaos, and the Madness of city life,[20]

---

18   N. J. Wade, 'The Original Spin Doctors—The Meeting of Perception and Insanity', *Perception*, 34(3), (2005), 253–60.

19   Sometimes referred to as William.

20   https://www.bbc.com/culture/article/20161213-how-bedlam-became-a-palace-for-lunatics (last accessed January 2023).

slowly began to crumble in the middle of London. Its palace-like appearance, it emerged, was underpinned by some inescapable structural flaws. The building's facade was so heavy that it cracked at the back – letting in wind and water any time it rained.[21] Rather symbolically, it had also been built too hastily to accommodate for rising levels of incarceration, on an unsteady foundation of rubble.[22] After standing for less than 150 years, the 'palace for lunatics' was torn down in 1815, to be rebuilt in Lambeth, South London. The only spatial remnant of the building is another blue tile, affixed to a wall outside Pizza Express in Finsbury Circus.

Regulating Madness

Despite the chaos and scandal that had racked 'new Bethlem', in the nineteenth century, the number of people committed to asylums skyrocketed, for a number of reasons. Firstly, the industrial revolution meant that Mad and disabled people could no longer work or be cared for in the home. Workers were sent into harsh factory conditions, where time pressure was immense, and people had little control over their working conditions – which was largely inhospitable to anyone who wasn't able-bodied/minded.[23] With these developments, family members of disabled and Mad people could also no longer be at home and care for their relatives. Relatedly, the Poor Law of 1834 stripped people in poverty of their financial support, and sent them into workhouses to prove their worth – an additional factor that meant

---

21   Ibid.

22   Ibid.

23   M. Oliver, 'The Politics of Disablement — New Social Movements', *The Politics of Disablement Critical Texts in Social Work and the Welfare State* (London: Palgrave, 1990).

that even the unemployed could no longer care for their Mad relatives.

Another significant reason behind the increase of Mad incarcerated people in the nineteenth century was the passing of two Asylum Acts, which first allowed, and later mandated, counties to establish their own publicly funded mental asylums. Since the asylums were being built, counties would find people to fill them. Alongside the Poor Laws, this legislation laid the foundations of the modern welfare state;[24] it was a way of *managing* poor, disabled and unruly bodyminds that could not be easily exploited for profit.[25] While Madness and disability had always existed up until this point, this marked a significant moment in the state officially *regulating*, *controlling* and *certifying* Madness and disability. Since counties were taking Mad people into their care en masse, Madness became something that had to be examined and signed off on by state institutions, rather than something that just . . . was. Its boundaries had to be hardened, measured and, crucially, proven to be so incompatible with work that people couldn't possibly labour in a factory. Therefore the line between Madness and sanity became dependent on the capitalist mode of production and managed by the state.

Treating people's morals

The institutions that were unfurling across each of Britain's counties in the nineteenth century were slightly different in nature to those that had come before. Influenced by the criticism that had snowballed in previous decades, nineteenth century institutions were adopting a new approach to care and

---

24 https://lrb.co.uk/podcasts-and-videos/podcasts/the-lrb-podcast/the-last-asylums (last accessed January 2023).

25 Ibid.

cure – something they termed 'moral treatment'. The implications of this name are suitably vague; is it that the treatment was more 'moral' than previous ones? Or that it was Mad people's morals that were being treated? In my mind, the answer is: a bit of both.

Moral treatment was foreshadowed by a few figures across Europe, including Philippe Pinel, who supposedly began 'freeing the insane from their chains' in France towards the end of the century prior, and the Quaker William Tuke, who had established an unconventional institution in York around the same time. At Tuke's asylum, people were also unchained, and there were no bars on the windows, since Tuke, like Pinel, advocated for 'gentler' forms of restraint, like the straitjacket. The institution was also incredibly domestic in its approach. The community was supposedly a 'family', the patients, 'like children', and the asylum's superintendent, a parental figure.[26] Residents had dinner with asylum managers and prayed with them. They were treated kindlier, and were encouraged to eat well, exercise and rest. These principles of moral treatment, which were not devised by doctors, but by Quakers, would soon become the dominant approach across all asylums.

Moral treatment was in some ways different, and in others it was a continuation of the approach that had come before. It was undoubtedly considered to be kinder – championed as a 'rational, humane and modern'[27] approach to Madness. But it was still a method of institutionalisation and control. Rather than acting upon people's bodies through physical discipline, moral treatment centred around the social concept of 'self-dis-

26   R. Porter, *Mind-forg'd Manacles: A History of Madness in England from the Restoration to the Regency* (Cambridge, MA: Harvard University Press, 1987).

27   A. Brigham, 'The moral treatment of insanity: 1847', *The American Journal of Psychiatry*, 151:6 Suppl, (1994), pp. 10–15.

cipline', encouraging patients to establish the regular habits and self-control that they had supposedly not gained in the home. Residents were, for example, given simple rewards for 'rational' behaviour, and encouraged to participate in everyday activities like manual labour, religious worship, painting, crafts and other preoccupations that might 'divert' people from their thoughts.[28] The institution also generally emphasised 'productive' activities. Residents might be expected to contribute to work like farming, dressmaking, baking, carpentry or the manufacturing of toys, shoes and books[29] – a form of forced labour that still takes place in some psychiatric institutions and prisons today. While it was argued that these preoccupations were about engaging and distracting the mind, they were still a not-so-subtle reminder that being exploitable is part of the definition of sanity.[30]

As a 'humane' reform, which reaped better outcomes than its predecessors,[31,32] moral treatment undoubtedly helped solidify asylums as the 'solution' to Madness in the public imagination. Simultaneously, expansion continued to spiral, in a similar fashion to the prison system today. As more asylums were built, more people would fill them – when they continued to expand to accommodate for this, they would once again become overrun.[33] By the end of the nineteenth century, there were more than 100,000 people living in county pauper asylums, all of which were 'compulsory' patients detained by the state, and

28   Ibid.

29   Ibid.

30   Porter, *Mind-forg'd Manacles*.

31   E. Shorter, *A History of Psychiatry: From the Era of the Asylum to the Age of Prozac* (New York: John Wiley & Sons, 1997).

32   J. Haslam, *Observations*, pp. 295–6.

33   Porter, 'Madness and society in England'.

were less likely to be released than prisoners.[34] Giant institutions like Colney Hatch Lunatic Asylum in Friern had more than 2,000 beds.[35]

While the increasingly bleak, deprived and sickening conditions during the industrial revolution undoubtedly contributed to extremely high rates of Madness and subsequent incarceration, this is hard to measure, because of how pliable and unstable the concept of Madness continued to be. Some terms were fluid, for example, the categories of 'mania' and 'melancholia', which most Mad people were sorted into, were being used differently across the country.[36] Other categories, like 'moral insanity', were used in some places and not at all in others. 'Dementia' didn't have the same meaning it has today – it could mean anything from a head injury to what is now described as psychosis. Even the term 'Madness' encompassed a wide range of mind/brain states, including conditions like syphilis of the brain and alcoholism. These inconsistencies were also reflected across the globe – with some asylums in the US listing arbitrary and politically laden reasons for incarceration like 'immoral life', 'politics' and 'novel reading'.[37] While this system of categorisation might seem clearly dubious today, these examples are not simply historical errors, which have now been supplanted by 'true' or 'natural' diagnoses. Rather, they reveal how diagnosis has long reflected shifting social and political expectations of populations.

---

34   T. Butler, 'The Making of the Mental Health Act, 1957–60', *Mental Health, Social Policy and the Law* (London: Palgrave Macmillan, 1985).

35   Shorter, *A History of Psychiatry*.

36   S. A. Hill and R. Laugharne, 'Mania, dementia and melancholia in the 1870s: admissions to a Cornwall asylum', *Journal of the Royal Society of Medicine*, 96:7, (2003), pp. 361–3.

37   B. M. Z. Cohen, *Psychiatric Hegemony: A Marxist Theory of Mental Illness* (London: Palgrave Macmillan, 2016).

As asylums ballooned in number and size, resembling ornate warehouses more than places of healing, their practices once again became extremely cold, impersonal and inhumane. New modes of physical suppression reared their heads, like the degrading padded cell and the administering of powerful sedatives. The physical environment inside the asylum walls once again deteriorated – people were sleeping without beds,[38] in conditions that closely resembled workhouses.[39] It became rapidly clear that the personalised 'affectionate attention',[40] which had been so central to the doctrine of moral treatment, was not the state's priority, nor was it a possibility in an era of increasing industrialisation, poverty, population growth and overcrowding. Pessimistic scientific theories emerged to diminish the state's responsibility for these failures, with 'degeneration theory' – the idea that Madness was incurable and was destined to deteriorate – becoming popular. While Pinel may have removed some people's chains, their metaphorical chains remained very much intact.

The birth of psychiatry

In the early twentieth century, the institution we recognise as 'psychiatry' began to assert its identity as a science and a medical specialism. Until this point, there had been 'Mad doctors', 'alienists' and 'asylum superintendents' – who managed Mad people in asylums. But they weren't organised in a coherent way, and

38 D. Budden, *A County Lunatic Asylum: The History of St. Matthew's Hospital* (Burntwood: St. Matthew's Hospital, Pharmacy Department, 1989), pp. 60–62.

39 E. Myers, 'Workhouse or asylum: The nineteenth century battle for the care of the pauper insane', *Psychiatric Bulletin*, 22:9, (1998), pp. 575–7.

40 W. C. Ellis, *A Treatise on the Nature, Symptoms, Causes, and Treatment of Insanity* (London: Holdsworth, 1838), pp. 6–7.

they were judged by many people as unscientific, and inferior to general doctors.

Around this time, the German psychiatrist Emil Kraepelin began to advance the idea that mental disorders were legitimate 'disease entities',[41] which could be categorised. He was influenced by the eugenicist, Francis Galton[42] (cousin to Charles Darwin), who felt that there was such a thing as a biologically 'normal mind'. During this period, Kraepelin broke mental disorders down into discrete disease categories like 'dementia praecox' (now known as schizophrenia), and 'manic depressive psychosis' (which became bipolar), and tried to cement the idea that they were biological in origin. Other psychiatrists joined the effort to bolster psychiatry as a medical specialism – for example, by doing experimental research, and advocating for it to be taught in universities.[43] The asylum system had, in a sense, now birthed a discipline, which prided itself as a science.

This scientific veneer would soon be reflected back by the asylum itself. In 1930, the Mental Treatment Act changed the name of asylums to 'mental hospitals'; and, following suit, 'attendants' became 'nurses', and 'lunatics' became 'patients'. While psychoanalysis and talking therapies were becoming more popular outside the asylum, people on the inside were subject to new painful physical interventions: insulin shock therapy, in which patients diagnosed as schizophrenic were induced into comas; lobotomies, which involved severing parts of the brain; and electroconvulsive therapy (ECT), in which seizures were induced by passing an electric current through the brain (patients were not given muscle relaxants, and so frequently broke bones). These treatments often had irreversible effects on

41   R. Porter, *Madness: A Brief History* (Oxford: Oxford University Press, 2002).

42   R. Chapman, *Empire of Normal* (London: Pluto Press, forthcoming).

43   Shorter, *A History of Psychiatry*.

the brain, but, similarly to the bloodletting and purging that took place two centuries prior, violence was veiled by the promise of cure, and now, the expertise and objectivity of medicine.

During the Second World War, mass atrocities were committed against asylum residents. In 1939, German psychiatrists participated in the selection process for the Nazi Aktion T-4 programme, which killed over 70,000 psychiatric patients via carbon monoxide gas.[44] Some professionals were unaware of what they were participating in, while others knew – one asylum even celebrated the cremation of its 10,000[th] patient with a bottle of beer for everyone in attendance.[45] By the end of the war, somewhere between 73 and 100% of people in Germany identified as schizophrenic had been either sterilised or killed.[46] In the shadow of the war, there was a shift from biological theories of Madness/Mental Illness, to psychoanalytic ones – which saw them as originating from the family and the social world, rather than an inevitable genetic defect within the brain.

Psychiatry in dissent

While the gay, Black and women's civil rights struggles picked up speed during the 1960s, there was another movement unfolding, which is largely forgotten in many political spaces today. The 'anti-psychiatry' movement, which contested psychiatric authority, was made up of a vast and nebulous constellation of critics of psychiatry from across the political spectrum. Anti-psychiatry was a complex and contentious struggle for two particular reasons: firstly, because it was primarily led by

---

44   E. F. Torrey and R. H. Yolken, 'Psychiatric genocide: Nazi attempts to eradicate schizophrenia', *Schizophrenia Bulletin*, 36:1, (2010), pp. 26–32.

45   Ibid.

46   Ibid.

psychiatrists themselves, who challenged some of the fundamental foundations of the discipline; but also, because many of the figures who are now most associated with the movement vehemently rejected the label of 'anti-psychiatry' altogether.

This is perhaps because the movement was made up of such a diverse range of political commitments. The psychiatrist Franco Basaglia, for example, was an anti-fascist who had been imprisoned for his political activity in Venice, during the Second World War. His criticism of psychiatry, which we will look at in Chapter 10, was therefore centred around the prison-like conditions in asylums. On the other end of the spectrum, the Hungarian psychiatrist Thomas Szasz was a right-wing libertarian, who believed that the concept of Mental Illness was a myth,[47] which led to some people being unfairly locked up in asylums, and prevented others from taking responsibility for their actions. Meanwhile, the Scottish psychiatrist, R. D. Laing (who flirted with Marxism but pulled away from it in later years), wanted to find *meaning* in Madness, for example, listening to the supposed 'ramblings' of people diagnosed with schizophrenia, to decipher their messages.[48] These thinkers had very different opinions on whether Mental Illness existed, and how we should approach it; but what united them was their criticism of the *very basis* of psychiatry,[49] and the asylum system from which it sprung. Other liberation movements took some interest in anti-psychiatry, during a period in which the label of Madness/Mental Illness

---

47   T. Szasz, The Myth of Mental Illness: Foundations of a Theory of Personal Conduct (New York, NY: Harper & Row, 1961).

48   R. D. Laing, *The Divided Self: An Existential Study in Sanity and Madness* (London: Tavistock Publications, 1969).

49   N. Crossley, 'R. D. Laing and the British anti-psychiatry movement: a socio-historical analysis', *Social Science & Medicine*, 47:7, (1998[1982]), pp. 877–89.

was applied to homosexuality and Black radicalism[50] (two issues
that we will return to in Chapters 3 and 7). In 1967, an event
called the Dialectics of Liberation Congress was held in London,
which brought together anti-psychiatrists like Laing and David
Cooper, and other radicals, like the Black power leader Stokely
Carmichael.[51]

As we saw during the controversy of 'new Bethlem', the phenomenon of professionals criticising asylums, and the treatment
of the Mad, was actually not new. The commonly voiced opinion
that distress should not be thought of as a physical illness had
all come before during the 'moral treatment' era. What was
relatively unusual was that during the same period, hospital
patients, or as they started to call themselves, 'psychiatric survivors', began to organise on a much larger scale than previous
centuries,[52] revolting against psychiatry too. In 1971, a group of
patients at Hartwood Hospital in Scotland established the first
'Mental Patients' Union', through which they started to make
demands to change their living conditions. Another union was
established at Paddington Day Hospital in London, for which
patients later established a headquarters in a Camden squat.
Mental Patients' Unions continued to spring up across the
country, as well as other groups like Campaign Against Psychiatric Oppression (CAPO), Survivors Speak Out, the Hearing Voices
Network and Community Organisation for Psychiatric Emer-
gencies (COPE). In Germany, a revolutionary group called the
Socialist Patients' Collective (SPK) formed, which attempted to

---

50   J. M. Metzl, *The Protest Psychosis: How Schizophrenia Became a Black Disease*
(London: Beacon Press, 2009).

51   R. Laing, D. Cooper, H. Marcuse, S. Carmichael, *The Dialectics of Liberation*
(London: Verso Books, 2015).

52   However, a small number of patients rights groups such as the Alleged Lunatics'
Friend Society had briefly sprung up in previous centuries.

situate mental and physical illness in the context of capitalism. Many of these groups attempted to take care and treatment into their own hands – for example, Hackney Mental Patients' Union let people in crisis crash in their squat, and SPK conducted 'group agitations', in which they tried to identify and remedy the material needs of patients. Each of these groups posed a radical challenge to individualised psychiatric control, emphasising collective care, political transformation and survivor agency.

Deinstitutionalisation: a partial revolution

It was clear, by the 1980s, that the institution of the asylum, and psychiatry more broadly, was losing public legitimacy. In Britain, more and more scandals regarding the treatment of patients were also getting out in the press, some of which resulted in inquiries. Governments were under pressure to listen to public criticism of the asylum system. I would argue, however, that they really chose to listen to the chill winds of the market.[53]

'Deinstitutionalisation', a programme of mass psychiatric hospital closure, saw the county asylums that had rapidly expanded across the country in the nineteenth century dismantled at a similar rate during the second half of the twentieth century. The closure of psychiatric institutions wasn't mandated by a left-wing government, or any leader who necessarily sympathised with patients and survivors themselves. Rather, deinstitutionalisation had been first called for by Enoch Powell, an early neoliberal politician, and taken up as a widespread policy by Prime Minister Margaret Thatcher in the 1980s. In the US, these developments were mirrored under Ronald Reagan. This might feel counter-intuitive – what stake did Conserva-

---

53   A. Scull, *Decarceration: Community Treatment and the Deviant - A Radical View* (London: Basil Blackwell, 1984).

tives have in closing mental hospitals? But, in fact, the closure of asylums chimed perfectly with neoliberal agendas, which saw many state institutions dismantled and privatised.

A policy called 'care in the community' was also introduced, transferring responsibility from hospitals onto families and local mental health services. This may all sound quite nurturing. However, in reality, many Mad/Mentally Ill people were moved out of punishing institutions, and into a punishing world. As was the case during the industrial revolution, their families still had to go to work, and Mad/Mentally Ill people were still largely excluded from the job market. It is unsurprising, therefore, that in the decades following deinstitutionalisation, the proportion of Mad/Mentally Ill houseless people and prisoners increased. Much to the anticipation of many people across history, the asylum era may have 'officially' come to an end, but the conditions of Mad/Mentally Ill people under capitalism had not been revolutionised. After centuries of violence, it seems clear to me that the transformation needed didn't start and end at the institution. We needed to transform our material conditions on the outside too – to transform the world.

Asylums in the rear-view mirror

In 2015, when construction was underway for the London Underground's Elizabeth Line, Crossrail workers discovered skeletons in the ground beneath Liverpool Street. It later came to light that they had unearthed a 'Bedlam burial site'[54] – a mass grave in which up to 20,000 people had been buried over

---

54   https://bbc.co.uk/news/uk-england-london-31800670 (last accessed January 2023).

a 150-year period spanning the plague.[55] Most of the remains retrieved had actually belonged to local people, who were buried in the churchyard next to Bethlem due to the overcrowding of other cemeteries.[56] However, some of the skeletons were those of Bethlem's 'lunatiks'.[57] Despite this slightly tangential relationship to the asylum itself, the media was briefly set ablaze with sensationalist stories about Bethlem, and the historic treatment of Mad people. The general gist of the coverage was: 'this is how it used to be'. But few asked: how is it *now*? Was there a true structural break between the past and the present?

Although the story of asylums may seem like a messy, distant history of competing ideas, approaches and reforms, there are a number of clear threads that can be extended from early Bethlem to today. For example, history makes clear that Madness/Mental Illnesses are not the stable, concrete or God-given categories that we are often led to believe they are. Whether we see Madness as an illness or a behaviour, biological or social, is also irrelevant to the fact that the Madness we recognise today was *constructed* in line with the demands of the capitalist system. The concrete, 'objective' line between Madness and sanity that we often take to be clear cut, only became necessary when the state needed to determine who could work, and who needed to be institutionalised. Like other constructs, this dividing line has also bent and redrawn itself across history, in line with changing social forces and ideologies of the time. This is an idea that we will return to

55   https://edition.cnn.com/2015/03/10/europe/bedlam-burial-ground (last accessed January 2023).

56   https://museumofthemind.org.uk/blog/those-bedlam-bones-again-1 (last accessed January 2023).

57   https://crossrail.co.uk/benefits/archaeology/bedlam-burial-ground-register (last accessed January 2023).

again and again throughout this book – how the categories of Mad/sane, sick/healthy are wobbly, messy and contextual.

While it is easy to look back on the systems of the past as uniquely villainous, we should actively bridge the gap between the logics of the past and those of today. Historic medical and psychiatric practices have almost always appealed to the idea of scientific objectivity or moral righteousness. 'Ordinary' people, who either went to gawk at Mad people in the eighteenth century, or excused these systems as they continued into the modern era, were also often guided by their own sense of morality, trust in medicine, or a belief that this was, unfortunately, how things had to be. One crucial thing that we can learn from the past is that no scientific or moral 'common sense' produces itself within a vacuum, free from the interference of the social systems we are embedded in. Today's 'objective' or 'rational' knowledge is also infused with values that we cannot see – for example, we still grapple with drugs and treatments that are painful or have deeply unpleasant side effects, even though we don't fully understand the science behind them.[58] The same logics continue, even if psychiatrists who tell their own history of the discipline might want us to believe otherwise.

It would also be premature to say that institutionalisation is simply a horror of the past, which has now been eradicated. Over 50,000 people are still detained under the Mental Health Act each year,[59] legislation that makes it possible to lock people up in psychiatric facilities without their consent. When people are hospitalised under section, many are still routinely subject

---

58   J. Moncrieff, R. E. Cooper, T. Stockmann, et al., 'The serotonin theory of depression: a systematic umbrella review of the evidence', *Mol Psychiatry* (2022).

59   https://digital.nhs.uk/data-and-information/publications/statistical/mental-health-act-statistics-annual-figures/2020-21-annual-figures (last accessed January 2023).

to abuse, forced treatment, restraint and other violations in bodily autonomy. Many other Mad/Mentally Ill people are now incarcerated in prisons. Rather symbolically, a number of asylums, for example, All Saints Asylum in Birmingham, have either been converted to prisons or now host prisons on the sites where they used to stand. And, as the historian Clair Wills has pointed out, as old mental hospitals closed, a more recent form of state incarceration began to expand across Britain.[60] Today, tens of thousands of people are detained in immigration removal centres each year in the UK. These people, like those kept in Victorian institutions, are still described as seeking 'asylum'.[61]

Refusing to look

Our society locked Mad people up because they became inconvenient to, and incompatible with, the social and economic order. They were swept out of public sight, only to be periodically gazed at as a morbid curiosity, or a cautionary tale. Their very existence was awkward – a taboo. For all of our talk about 'awareness raising' and 'speaking out' about mental health, our approach to the history of Madness is shrouded in awkwardness and taboo too.

Growing up on the outskirts of North London, I often heard gossip about the luxury flats on a nearby complex called Princess Park Manor, in Friern Barnet. The towering mansion, set on 30 acres of private parkland, housed *X Factor* stars, boy band members and professional footballers.[62] What you wouldn't

---

60   https://lrb.co.uk/podcasts-and-videos/podcasts/the-lrb-podcast/the-last-asylums (last accessed January 2023).

61   Ibid.

62   https://independent.co.uk/property/house-and-home/the-new-cast-of-neighbours-why-the-bling-brigade-is-flocking-to-a-former-asylum-in-north-london-7546090.html (last accessed January 2023).

find on the manor's website, or on any of its property listings, however, was the fact that the building was formerly Colney Hatch Lunatic Asylum, what was once the largest asylum in Europe. This revelation is by no means unusual. Asylums are truly all around us, everywhere in Britain, and their buildings are still used to capitalist ends. Many have been sold off to become luxury hotels, homes, even gyms and spas – with their ornate, historic architecture serving as a key selling point. You can find converted asylums at Hotel du Vin in Edinburgh, The Bannatyne Spa Hotel in Hastings, The Residence luxury apartments in Kent, Parklands Manor apartments in Wakefield, Belgrove Place apartments in Ipswich, The Galleries apartments in Essex, the Repton Park Virgin Active gym in Essex, St Bernard's Gate apartments in Ealing, and Royal Earlswood Park apartments in Surrey, to name a few. But estate agents and businesses know that no one wants to talk about it – to acknowledge this reality of Britain's history.

If anything, they help us shut it off, and cast it further out of sight. When St. George's Hospital in Wiltshire was being converted into apartments, some people reported that they felt uneasy on site, prompting developers to call in a spiritualist to clear what was described as 'inappropriate energy'.[63] But how possible is it, really, to clear this energy, when we are unwilling to confront the foundations of our approach to mental health today? Or when we preach the importance of 'opening up' about depression and anxiety, but remain silent on diagnoses like schizophrenia, bipolar, dissociative identity disorder (DID), or other experiences that are stigmatised as *truly* Mad? How can we feel at ease when we continue to use scary stories and episodes of *The Simpsons* to manage our anxieties about what our society

---

63   https://gazetteandherald.co.uk/news/7369858.expert-called-in-to-exorcise-bad-energy/ (last accessed January 2023).

has done with Mad people, and what it continues to do with them? When the word 'Bedlam' has become a flippant descriptor of chaos or disorder – but we still stumble to find words to describe the psychiatric unit down the street, or refuse to talk about it at all?

When we talk about mental health 'awareness' today, that should mean confronting our discomfort, and genuinely opening our eyes to the reality of Madness in Britain. When you start to look, it isn't hard to see it; it is in every county, in every community, in the mental health system, on the plaques and in the buildings we walk among, it is in the ground beneath our feet.

Chapter 2

'Knowing' mental health today

This chapter contains a mention of suicide.

A few years ago, I gained a funded place on a two-day Mental Health First Aid training course through work. It was the sort of intensive crash course in mental health awareness that has increasingly grown in popularity in recent years, with 660,000 adults now trained by Mental Health First Aid England, specifically.[1] Throughout the course, we learned about common mental health problems, their symptoms, how to spot them, and practical skills, like how to support someone who's experiencing a panic attack. The memory from the course that has stuck with me the most, however, was an exercise that was intended to help us better understand what it feels like to hear voices (medically understood as a symptom of psychosis).

For a few minutes, we were instructed to step away from our horseshoe-shaped table, to find a quiet place with a few others, and for one participant (let's say, Person A) to whisper down a long, cardboard wrapping paper tube, into the ear of Person B. Then, Person B would have to try to hold a conversation with Person C, while ignoring the distracting voice in their ear. The goal was to simulate the experience of psychosis – and to demon-

---

1   https://mhfaengland.org/mhfa-centre/blog/progress-in-a-pandemic-mental-health-first-aid-in-numbers/ (last accessed January 2023).

strate how hard it is to concentrate on a 'real' conversation when you are hearing voices. People laughed, struggled and despaired their way through the exercise. Then, we went back to the table, and back to our lives.

At the time, I felt like I gained something concrete from the exercise, but reflecting on the experience, years later, I also wonder what I lost. I understood the point of the exercise – for people to put themselves in 'another person's shoes' and think about an experience that seemed abstract to them. But it also affirmed the idea that a person can understand the experience of voice-hearing by isolating a superficial 'symptom' and trying to 'immersively' experience it. In doing so, we stripped voice-hearing of context. For example, many people who hear voices don't become distressed by them simply because they're *distracting*, but because of how the experience of hearing voices is constructed in our society.[2] For others, voice-hearing might be distressing because their voices say frightening or disturbing things.[3] The bottom line is that everyone who hears voices will have a different experience. By suggesting that attendees can understand voice-hearing from this experience in a stale, university seminar room, we suggest that it is something we can definitively *know*.[4]

But how 'knowable' is mental health really? By 'knowable', I mean, how easy is it to package it up, to objectively describe or quantify it, and to quickly tokenise it for other people to under-

---

2   https://news.stanford.edu/2014/07/16/voices-culture-luhrmann-071614/ (last accessed January 2023).

3   https://mentalhealth.org.uk/explore-mental-health/a-z-topics/hearing-voices (last accessed January 2023).

4   It is worth noting that this exercise was originally developed by the Hearing Voices movement (which is made up of people with lived experience of hearing voices and seeing visions). However, in this instance, it was largely stripped of its context and critical edge.

stand? Societally, I sense a rush to make mental health digestible – we see it everywhere from 'awareness-raising' campaigns, to self-care narratives, to traditional psychiatry. But this approach ultimately aligns with capitalist principles of extraction and commodification – made starker in the context of workshops that extract knowledge from Mad/Mentally Ill people and sell it to employers and institutions. It is also underpinned by a colonial and enlightenment mindset, which sees Madness/Mental Illness as territory we can discover, map and conquer.

As mental health is packaged and presented to us by supposedly 'all-knowing' experts, it is important to scrutinise the messages they pass on. We should also interrogate the very idea that we can objectively know and conquer mental health knowledge – and question whether this is something we should be striving to do at all.

The age of awareness

There are many reasons why we might try to understand mental health with certainty. We currently find ourselves in the midst of what has been described as a global mental health crisis. Two in every five GP appointments are about mental health,[5] and every 10 seconds, someone in England or Wales calls the emotional support line Samaritans.[6] In the same regions, suicide is the leading cause of death in men under 50.[7] Shortly before the

5   https://mind.org.uk/news-campaigns/news/40-per-cent-of-all-gp-appointments-about-mental-health/ (last accessed January 2023).

6   https://samaritans.org/support-us/why-we-need-your-help/ (last accessed January 2023).

7   https://ons.gov.uk/peoplepopulationandcommunity/healthandsocialcare/causesofdeath/articles/leadingcausesofdeathuk/2001to2018 (last accessed January 2023). Women, however, are more likely to experience suicidal thoughts and attempt suicide, as found by Canetto and Sakinofsky, 1998 and McManus et al., 2016.

Covid-19 pandemic, one in 10 British adults were said to experience some form of depression, with one in six adults in England prescribed an antidepressant over the course of a year.[8] To me and many others, these statistics and the realities that underlie them are urgent and overwhelming.

It makes sense, therefore, that we find ourselves in a race to know and understand mental health, to – like an emergency grab bag – package up need-to-know mental health knowledge in the form of 'first aid' and crisis management. I have often, in situations where I have been supporting others, found great solace and instruction in being given a document or a training and being told *how to spot it and what to do*. The ability to label, fix and control experiences that feel nonsensical and chaotic – to give them clearer contours that I can hold on to and handle – has felt reassuring and stabilising. Equally, I have witnessed moments where authoritative knowledge and rigid certainty has been insufficient or even harmful. For example, while one person may want to be touched or held while experiencing a panic attack, another person might find this actively distressing. Further differences also crop up across cultural contexts. We can't always superimpose our knowledge on others, because we cannot always be certain.

Recent decades have seen an upsurge in calls for, and activities described as, 'mental health awareness'. Awareness is championed by a huge range of actors, from government figures, to medical professionals, to celebrities, to large mental health charities. Mental health awareness is rarely defined by its biggest proponents, but it generally centres around three key principles: encouraging people to see mental health as 'important', providing people with information so they can 'spot the

8   https://gov.uk/government/publications/prescribed-medicines-review-report/ prescribed-medicines-review-summary (last accessed January 2023).

signs' and go to services for different mental health concerns, and 'reducing stigma' towards Madness/Mental Illness. Awareness sometimes comes from the top down, for example, when experts are called in to tell us the symptoms of various mental health problems. Other times, the onus of disseminating information falls on people themselves, with an emphasis on Mad/Mentally Ill people making personal disclosures to others, or 'reaching out' to services for help.

Awareness campaigns often describe mental health in reference to its normality and familiarity – through phrases like 'we all have mental health'.[9,10] These communications frequently transform subjective and taboo experiences into tokens that can be digested and understood. One clear example of this is the use of numbers; the phrase *one in four*[11] (the number of adults who have been reported to experience a psychiatric disability every year) has become a sort of received wisdom, which succinctly quantifies the scale of the crisis. But what do we lose from this kind of simplification? Can a statistic, clear and repeatable as it may be, ever do justice to the deeply personal and indescribable experience of, for example, feeling suicidal?

Other campaigns have used familiar metaphors to make the slippery concept of Madness more concrete. In the 2010s, the World Health Organisation (WHO) and the mental health charity SANE used the concept of a 'black dog' to symbolise depression.[12,13] The motif, made famous by former Prime

---

9   https://annafreud.org/schools-and-colleges/resources/we-all-have-mental-health-animation-teacher-toolkit/ (last accessed January 2023).

10   https://mentalhealth.org.uk/explore-mental-health/about-mental-health (last accessed January 2023).

11   S. Ginn and J. Horder, '"One in four" with a mental health problem: the anatomy of a statistic', *BMJ*, 344:e1302, (2012).

12   https://youtube.com/watch?v=XiCrniLQGYc (last accessed January 2023).

13   https://sane.org.uk/news-campaigns-media/campaigns/black-dog-campaign (last accessed January 2023).

Minister Winston Churchill, successfully transformed a diagnosis that is shrouded in mystery and complexity, into a (quite
literally) cuddly and familiar object, which can be handled,
'tamed' or even trained into submission. Other discussions have
used the image of a dark cloud, a broken leg, a war or a parasite,
to make depression visible and knowable. Again, it is not that
these comparisons are always concretely inaccurate, but that
they are, in their very nature, simplifying.

Beyond statistics and metaphors, the 'awareness' push often
attempts to make mental health more friendly and familiar by
presenting it on 'normal', non-threatening people. For example,
campaigns, bestselling mental health memoirs, fiction, television shows, and other discussions of mental health in the
mainstream often present Madness/Mental Illness through the
bodyminds of white, middle class, able-bodied and 'recovered'
people. They may not tick all of these boxes, but they invariably
fit our societal expectations of 'respectability', the opposite of
criminality or threat to the social order. The underlying message
is that there is nothing to be afraid of here. As part of this assim-
ilationist approach, certain mental health problems are also
prioritised as more recognisable, safe and 'knowable' than others.
Much of the time, the phrase 'mental health' in itself functions
as a sort of colloquial shorthand for depression and anxiety. As
concerns that we are all seen to have proximity to, and are generally not demonised as dangerous or threatening, depression
and anxiety are framed as legible, human and familiar. In 2017,
Emma Simkin wrote about this idea in *Blueprint*:

> [When I was diagnosed with depression,] almost all of my
> friends and family had either experienced depression them-
> selves, or known someone who had, so would relate to my
> experiences with kindness and sympathy . . . A few years

down the line, with a new diagnosis of bipolar disorder, my experiences have been very different. As part of the package of bipolar, sometimes I suffer from more unpalatable mental health issues, such as delusions. Tell someone you're feeling low and struggling to get out of bed, and aside from offering kindness and support, no one really bats an eyelid. Tell the same person that you think that motorway signs are giving you hidden messages about the secrets of time, and they look at you like you've just grown three heads or murdered a puppy.[14]

Those who are 'disruptive', whose Madness/Mental Illness cannot be easily realigned with capitalist metrics of exploitability, are excluded from the project of mental health awareness. This helps bolster the idea that they are unsalvageable, and therefore legitimate targets for incarceration and other forms of state violence. This two-tier system is by no means a new phenomenon; all throughout the asylum era there were plenty of people that were seen to have low-level 'neuroses' that were treated via spa visits or psychoanalysts rather than institutionalisation.[15] Meanwhile, those viewed as more unproductive and threatening to the social order have historically been targeted and vanished from society. Even Winston Churchill, who used the 'black dog' as a euphemism for his depression, called for the introduction of forced labour camps for 'mental defectives'.[16] People viewed as 'really Mad' have always experienced the sharp end of sanism – the oppression of anyone perceived to be insane. By largely focusing on the familiarity of depression and anxiety,

---

14   https://blueprintzine.com/portfolio/mental-illness-exists-beyond-depression-and-anxiety-why-dont-we-talk-about-it/ (last accessed January 2023).

15   Shorter, *A History of Psychiatry*.

16   Hansard, *Parliamentary Debates*, 10 February 1911.

awareness-raising has failed to respond to the oppression of those who cannot assimilate, and are seen as unpredictable, or 'unknowable' within Western capitalist societies.

Depoliticising mental health knowledge

The push towards awareness frequently obscures the broader politics of mental health. In awareness narratives, the knowledge we are provided with often looks at mental health as something that takes place in a social vacuum, focusing on the level of the individual. To return to the hearing voices exercise in the Mental Health First Aid course, it presented psychosis as a negative experience primarily *because* of an internal symptom, rather than looking at the sanism that people with these experiences face in the wider world. This overlooks the fact that, to be 'psychotic', and to hear voices, is often seen as the ultimate and most dangerous form of Madness/Mental Illness – it has led people to be barred from employment, brutalised by police, imprisoned, institutionalised, and a host of other structural harms. The academic Alison Kafer has criticised this kind of individualism in other disability awareness workshops – for example, in exercises where people wear blindfolds or use wheelchairs to simulate vision or mobility impairment. She writes: 'Although these kinds of exercises are intended to reduce fears and misperceptions about disabled people . . . [absent] are discussions about disability rights and social justice; disability is depoliticised, presented more as nature than culture.'[17]

When awareness narratives do look at culture, the concept of 'stigma' is often deployed in particularly apolitical ways. The concept of stigma centres around the notion that a person or

---

17   A. Kafer, *Feminist, Queer, Crip* (Bloomington: Indiana University Press, 2013).

group of people are 'spoiled' by an undesirable mark or characteristic. However, stigma doesn't just come from one place, and it can vary depending on context. We see contradictory statements about stigma all the time when people talk about mental health, for example, some people say they experience stigma because they take medication, others say they experience stigma because they *don't* take medication. In actuality, both groups are experiencing sanism because of their supposedly spoiled identity. Similarly, decades ago, there was a mainstream 'stigma' against having to see a therapist, but today, many argue that there is a stigma against *not* going to therapy. We therefore lose something when we discuss stigma as a blanket or universal concept that always operates in one direction. Stigma can spring up in lots of different places and can, on the face of it, appear to be contradictory.

Anti-stigma campaigners usually place the onus of tackling stigma on individuals, in two specific ways. Firstly, they suggest that people who hold stigmatising beliefs need to gain access to better knowledge, and educate themselves. They also suggest that people who experience any kind of mental distress should educate others. Both of these approaches see stigma as something that emerges organically from people, by either perpetuating it through bigoted attitudes and beliefs, or by sustaining it through personal secrecy.

We are often encouraged to 'bust stigma' by personally disclosing our mental health struggles to others. The suggestion that we must 'open up' or 'speak out' – which is often discussed in similar terms to the queer notion of 'coming out' – often implies that if we do this, we can normalise mental distress. This places responsibility for eradicating sanism on the very people who experience it. This may be dangerous for marginalised groups, including those whose diagnoses are most stigmatised, and those with less

43

societal power. While celebrities may in some contexts receive a positive reaction for being vulnerable about their mental health, a mother speaking to a social worker may see her children taken away.[18] As we will discuss in more detail in Chapter 9, 'opening up' about mental health can also see people locked up or harmed by police or by mental health professionals. In our current conditions, disclosure is simply not always safe.

The individualism of mental health awareness also trickles into our understandings of cure. Mental health awareness places responsibility for 'fixing' Madness/Mental Illness on individuals, by suggesting that if people have the correct knowledge about symptoms and how to address them, we can then solve this crisis among ourselves. The knowledge we are given to name and describe our struggles is usually psychiatric knowledge, which we will come to later in this chapter. Meanwhile, cure is framed as a clear and steady path, as long as we are willing to try going to health services, taking our medication, paying for therapy, practising self-care, taking up mindfulness, eating better, getting regular exercise, having an active social life – or anything else on the expanding list of practices that are promised to help us recover. While many of these things may make people feel better, an exclusive focus on these individual actions overlooks the fact that they don't work for everyone; and the road to 'recovery' is rocky, complex or even impossible for many of us in our current conditions. It frames ongoing distress as a personal failure to self-discipline or seek out appropriate services, rather than acknowledging the structural conditions that also dictate our lives. This approach aligns perfectly with neoliberal ideology, which emphasises free-market competition, decreased state spending, and increased personal responsibility.

18   I. Tyler and T. Slater, 'Rethinking the sociology of stigma', *The Sociological Review* 66, pp. 721–43.

Telling people to simply reach out to services, in particular, overwrites the knowledge of lots of Mad/Mentally Ill people, who already know about what is available to them. One million people sit on an NHS mental health waiting list,[19] and millions of others cannot gain access to resources because they are not considered to be the 'right kind of sick'. Meanwhile, many psychiatric survivors have had traumatising experiences within mental health services – how can 'more awareness' help them? Others bounce from one service to another, into the community and back again, with little improvement in their wellbeing. The journalist Hannah Jane Parkinson has articulated this frustration, writing:

> It isn't a bad thing that we are all talking more about mental health; it would be silly to argue otherwise. But this does not mean it is not infuriating to come home from a secure hospital, suicidal, to a bunch of celebrity awareness-raising selfies and thousands of people saying that all you need to do is ask for help – when you've been asking for help and not getting it.[20]

Awareness raising is by no means straightforwardly harmful or negative in itself. Many people, including myself, have benefited from conversations about one another's experiences. However, awareness-raising still largely diagnoses the mental health crisis as stemming from the faulty knowledge and behaviours of Mad/ Mentally Ill people and their loved ones. It also centres knowledge that reaffirms the status quo. A more liberating form of awareness would need to go beyond an individualised frame-

19 https://theguardian.com/society/2022/oct/10/nhs-mental-health-patients-wait-times (last accessed January 2023).
20 https://theguardian.com/society/2018/jun/30/nothing-like-broken-leg-mental-health-conversation (last accessed January 2023).

work, address our material conditions, and also account for our diverse and varied ways of thinking about mental health. For now, when we encounter awareness campaigns, it is always worth asking: what *exactly* are they trying to make us aware of?

The false promise of psychiatric knowledge

Psychiatry, beyond all other approaches to mental health, offers us the false yet reassuring promise and comfort of 'knowing'. For anyone looking to definitively conquer and understand mental health, psychiatric knowledge has a unique allure. Unlike the messy and subjective knowledge held by you or me, psychiatry claims to be objective, ordered and definitive.

Many doctors and psychiatrists use a tool published by the American Psychiatric Association (APA) called the Diagnostic and Statistical Manual of Mental Disorders (DSM) – which contains a list of Mental Illness categories and criteria that professionals can use to diagnose them ('diagnostic' criteria). The first and second editions of the DSM (released in the mid-twentieth century) were mainly informed by psychoanalysis, and saw 'mental disorder' as a spectrum, with each person's place on this spectrum influenced by social factors like unconscious drives, early childhood experiences and family dynamics.[21] However, in 1980, after the anti-psychiatry movement threatened psychiatry's legitimacy, the APA completely revolutionised the DSM, attempting to make it much more scientific in its approach.[22,23]

21 A. V. Horwitz, 'DSM - I and DSM – II', *Encyclopedia of Clinical Psychology*, eds R. L. Cautin and S. O. Lilienfeld, (2014).

22 A. J. Lewis, '"We are certain of our own insanity": Antipsychiatry and the gay liberation movement, 1968–1980', *Journal of the History of Sexuality*, 25:1, (2016). pp. 83–113.

23 R. Mayes, and A. V. Horwitz, 'DSM-III and the revolution in the classification of mental illness', *Journal of the History of the Behavioral Sciences*, 41:3, (2005), pp. 249–67.

It would now centre around Emil Kraepelin's suggestion (discussed in the previous chapter) that mental disorders were completely separate disease entities. Rather than existing on a spectrum, the DSM-3 tried to sort disorders into hard categories, which were supposedly biologically distinct from the 'normal' population.

Today, the DSM contains nearly 300 'mental disorders' (almost three times the number in the first edition) complete with a list of symptoms for each disorder. It aims to be practical, medical and certain, avoiding ambiguity and the subjective judgements of either practitioners or people themselves. Like other forms of medical diagnosis, the DSM opts for seemingly universal categories that are often applied across people, cultures and contexts[24] – like obsessive compulsive disorder (OCD), borderline personality disorder (BPD), and bipolar disorder. Similarly to the psychosis workshop exercise, the biological psychiatry of the DSM understands Madness/Mental Illness mostly on the level of disease symptoms, which should be viewed and addressed at surface level, often via chemical intervention. The 'problem' of Madness/Mental Illness is located in our individual bodyminds alone.

It is no coincidence that this biological psychiatric conception of Mental Illness became dominant in 1980, as neoliberal leaders like Margaret Thatcher and Ronald Reagan took office. Neoliberalism saw the privatisation of major businesses and cuts to state welfare, in favour of an emphasis on 'individual responsibility'. These leaders attempted to normalise the idea that the state was no longer responsible for us, rather, we were responsible for our own misfortune. The cultural theorist Mark Fisher noticed the link between neoliberal ideology and the changing

---

24 The fifth edition of the DSM made changes to allegedly incorporate 'a greater cultural sensitivity' – however, diagnoses are still applied across cultures in practice.

face of psychiatry, describing the shift towards individual illness framings during this period as just another form of privatisation: the privatisation of *stress*.[25] Fisher saw biological psychiatry as politically convenient to neoliberal capitalism, because it pinned distress on our brains in the form of 'chemical imbalances', rather than our social or material conditions. If we look at, for example, the framing of the workers' struggle since the dawn of neoliberalism, we can see evidence of this 'privatisation'. Over recent decades, strike days have fallen while working days lost to 'stress-related illness' have skyrocketed.[26] Biological psychiatry has provided us with a lens of analysis that ignores political disorder in favour of individual disorder.

The limits of scientific 'truth'

Psychiatric knowledge is also frequently damaging because of the dominance and power it holds in society. It is positioned as *expert* knowledge – bolstered by the institutional authority of science and medicine – and is therefore seen as more legitimate than knowledge that comes from people without power. This means that doctors and psychiatrists gain a monopoly on truth. They can diagnose and label us as they see fit, and override our knowledge of ourselves, or culturally derived knowledge. These decisions are also backed by the law. This power stems from the fact that, like the rest of medicine, psychiatry is seen to reveal internal, apolitical and ahistorical truths about our bodyminds, when, in actuality, its claims are socially and historically contextual, and closely tangled up in the demands of capitalist society.

---

25   M. Fisher, *Capitalist Realism: Is There No Alternative?* (Winchester, UK: Zero books, 2009).

26   https://theguardian.com/society/2016/feb/14/workplace-stress-hans-selye (last accessed January 2023).

Psychiatry's illnesses represent a production line approach to knowledge – they are framed not as *one subjective* way of knowing, but *the objective* way of knowing.

While we should resist this monolithic approach, we will also find problems with any alternative approach that attempts to make authoritative, blanket statements about the true, internal or scientific nature of mental health. For example, for professionals who, contrastingly, want to take a social approach to mental health, there is sometimes a temptation to follow in the tradition of the right wing anti-psychiatrist Thomas Szasz (discussed in the previous chapter), who believed that Mental Illness was not 'real' biological illness, but rather, an entirely social phenomenon.[27] Szasz pointed out that there was no evidence of biomarkers (physical markers, like genes or hormones) for Mental Illness, and so argued that they weren't 'objectively real', like physical illnesses were.

This argument runs into many pitfalls, but here we should focus on its fundamental approach to knowledge. Like psychiatric knowledge, this approach creates problems because it still uses physical medicine as the benchmark for objective truth.[28] It uses a medical argument – that there are currently no biomarkers for Mental Illness – to make an authoritative statement about how Mad/Mentally Ill people must understand themselves. This props up medicine's monopoly on knowledge and strips agency from people with lived experience. In fact, the same biomarker argument is often used to discount the experiences of people with physical conditions like fibromyalgia and myalgic encephalomyelitis/chronic fatigue syndrome (ME/CFS). In all this, there is very little room for people to craft their own subjective

27   T. Szasz, *The Myth of Mental Illness: Foundations of a Theory of Personal Conduct* (New York, NY: Harper & Row, 1961).

28   Sedgwick, *PsychoPolitics*.

meanings about their bodyminds, and to acknowledge all illness as something that is subjectively and socially experienced; not an objective category that can only be spoken into existence by Western medicine.

The same goes for arguments that sometimes spring up on the left, which suggest that Madness/Mental Illness is always caused by capitalism, oppression and other types of trauma. Of course, our political world vastly shapes our suffering. However, arguments that Madness/Mental Illness is *only* social overlook the fact that the 'biological versus social' is an artificial binary. There is no social without the biological and no biological without the social; social experiences are inscribed on our physical bodyminds, to be once again socially interpreted. To argue that Madness/Mental Illness is only caused by social factors also discounts the embodied experiences of many people. Sometimes suffering may feel more 'bodily', internal, random, messy, spontaneous or unknowable – in ways that we cannot always neatly trace to social triggers. We might believe they are drug, hormone or otherwise physically induced. They may be linked to other mental or physical disabilities. It is up to us to make sense of our own experiences – no professional, universalising philosophy or scientific theory should be able to dictate how we think about ourselves or what language we may use.

Different ways of knowing

Due to their position as 'experts', psychologists, psychiatrists, therapists, charities, academics, and other people in positions of power have always dominated the production of mental health knowledge. In the asylum era, professionals extracted knowledge from Mad/Mentally Ill people through studying and experimenting on them. Today, their knowledge is frequently co-opted, sometimes in professional forums where they are asked to represent the monolithic 'service user voice'. However, Mad/Mentally Ill people are still, paradoxically, often seen as incapable of knowledge production, because they are barred from 'rationality' and 'sanity'. They are framed as inherently illegitimate 'knowers' – something the philosopher Miranda Fricker has described as 'epistemic injustice'.[29] As a result of this injustice, people with lived experience have been systematically denied the ability to describe and narrate their own experiences as they see fit.

Taking seriously the knowledge of people who experience Madness/Mental Illness involves changing our approach to knowledge. We must uproot our assumptions and centre knowledge 'from below' – which often contradicts that of charities, medical institutions and other professional experts. For example, since its early days, the psychiatric survivor movement has seen the creation of harm reduction guides to psychiatric drugs,[30] written by and for people who actually have lived experience of them, and may have been misled or harmed by professionals. This type of knowledge stems from our embodied realities of moving through the world as people seen to be Mad/Mentally Ill. These realities are, by their very definition, subjective, fugitive and plural – they are scattered across contexts and cannot be unified to form one, definitive truth.

Questioning the way that we 'know' mental health doesn't involve rejecting all current knowledge, or resisting the pursuit of knowledge in the first place. Rather, it is about finding new ways to orient ourselves towards knowledge. This involves

---

29 M. Fricker, *Epistemic Injustice: Power and the Ethics of Knowing* (New York: Oxford University Press, 2007).

30 http://willhall.net/files/ComingOffPsychDrugsHarmReductGuide2Edonline.pdf (last accessed January 2023).

scrutinising and disrupting how power and capital shape our understanding of 'truth'. But it also means relinquishing the possibility of a final truth. We should resist the urge to authoritatively declare what mental health is and how we must know it. Politicising mental health does not demand having any sort of scientific or objective theory of what Mental Illness/Madness truly *is*.[31] This question is a distraction – it hinges on the troublesome notion of an objective scientific reality – and can never yield a final or satisfying answer.

The activist Jonah Bossewitch has argued that, in our mental health politics, we need to move towards an 'epistemological' approach.[32] By this, he means that we should not battle one another over how we *must know* mental health, but instead, embrace the infinite ways *that we might know it*. People think about and politicise their mental experiences differently. But these ideas do not necessarily have to be in competition. On the contrary, we can hold them together in solidarity. I also want us to be able to admonish the mindset of the omniscient scientist or investigator, looking to uncover and point towards a neat 'answer'. Instead, it is important to be able to sit with multiple, contradictory knowledges. How, for example, can we *know* a tree? Through poetry – by creatively describing one? Through a roleplay – by pretending to be one? Through art – by painting a beautiful picture of one? Or perhaps through biology, mathematics, photography, gardening, smell, or maybe touch? There is no *one way*.

Crucial to this approach is humility, which means questioning our own assumptions, and always remaining open to the idea

31 I adopt this position after Beatrice Adler-Bolton and Artie Vierkant in their book, *Health Communism* (London and New York: Verso, 2022).

32 J. Bossewitch, *The Mad Underground: A New Wave of Mad Resistance with Jonah Bossewitch* [video] Institute for the Development of Human Arts, (n.d.).

that we may be wrong.[33] We must be prepared to find knowledge in all kinds of places, not just a textbook or a seminar room. We must also accept the things we cannot know, resisting the often-oppressive urge to forcibly dominate, control and explain other people's suffering. The scientist and community organiser Ayesha Khan writes: 'colonial logic cannot fathom that there are many aspects of the universe that we as humans are unable to fully understand.'[34] This is something I think about a lot – how we are surrounded by seemingly invisible ultraviolet light and infrared waves that other species can perceive; how other creatures on this earth navigate the world through smell, echolocation or other modes of understanding that are completely alien to us; how experience and memory are subjective; how over 80% of the ocean is unexplored;[35] how an even greater proportion of the universe is a mystery to all of us; how our bodyminds are really a mystery too; and how you can never really know my experience and I can never really know yours. This can feel overwhelming, but it also pushes us to accept intangibility, ambivalence, strangeness, and the fact that there will always be things that there are no words for.

Ultimately, we cannot ever definitively know mental health, and so many of the ways we currently try to know it are restricted, oppressive or depoliticising. They represent but a sliver of what is actually possible – and when we see these as the only options, we narrow the imagination. Therefore, I don't want to dictate what we should think about mental health – on the contrary,

33 I borrow this idea from the psychiatric survivor Rachel Rowan Olive: https://soundcloud.com/national-elf-service/rachel-rowan-olive (last accessed January 2023).

34 https://wokescientist.substack.com/p/humans-are-not-separate-from-nature (last accessed January 2023).

35 https://ncei.noaa.gov/news/seabed-2030-map-gaps (last accessed January 2023).

I want to open up and point towards the boundless political possibilities of thinking and knowing and being. This task is something we have to balance with the urgency of our pain and suffering. But it can also show us new ways to move through it.

Chapter 3

Mental health in a maddening world

Freud and Adler and even the cosmic Jung did not think of the Negro in all their investigations. – Frantz Fanon

This chapter contains a mention of sexual abuse and discussions of suicide.

If we want to politicise illness and suffering, we cannot accept the idea that it is a biological lottery that snakes its way through society, randomly taking hold of our brain chemistry with no rhyme or reason. Suffering follows the political contours of our lives. As the climate crisis accelerates and economic crises become more frequent, we are not short of possible explanations for the global surge in mental distress. It also follows that mental distress affects us unevenly, counter to mainstream narratives that tell us that 'mental health does not discriminate'.

Our mental health cannot be disentangled from the intertwined systems of white supremacy, ableism, gendered oppression, imperialism and capitalism. All forms of what we call 'illness' or suffering interact with the political world – a world that is particularly deadly for certain bodyminds. Therefore, while we might all be being driven Mad, some of us are inevitably made Madder than others. When I say the world makes some of us Madder than others, this statement has two slightly distinct yet overlapping meanings. Firstly, the structures of our society make life less bearable for us – we are more likely to be anxious, traumatised and in despair. But I also mean that particular marginalised groups are more likely to be *categorised* or *labelled* as Mad. As we have established, Madness/Mental Illness are concepts that have been constructed in line with our ability to meet the capitalistic demands of our society. But they are also constructed alongside systems like gender, race and colonisation.

Then, different domains of oppression will also impact our experiences of mental health services and treatment. Whether you are poor, Black, a woman, a trans person, a disabled person, or a migrant, your identity will, to some extent, dictate how your distress is treated. It determines whether you are taken seriously, the type of care you have access to, whether you are treated violently or even killed when seeking mental healthcare. Therefore, when we talk about mental health and oppression, we need to account for these multiple realities: how the world *drives* us Mad, how the world comes to *categorise* us as Mad, and then, how the world *responds* to our Madness.

The colour of Madness[1]

How we are racialised in the world has serious impacts on our bodyminds. Race sees people sorted into socially significant categories like employable or unemployable, trustworthy or criminal, legal or illegal, intelligent or unintelligent, beautiful or ugly, exploiter or exploited, coloniser or colonised, rich or poor. People who are not read as white accumulate small and large bruises as we simply try to move through the world: we are more

[1] I borrow this phrase from Rianna Walcott and Samara Linton's book of the same name: *The Colour of Madness: Mental Health and Race in Technicolour* (London: Pan Macmillan, 2022).

likely to live in poverty, to be subject to policing and its violence, to be incarcerated, to be deprived of knowledge about our histories, to experience discrimination at work, and to develop particular physical illnesses. Accounting for each of these forms of violence, the scholar Ruth Wilson Gilmore defines racism as a force that makes us more vulnerable to premature death.[2]

When it comes to mental health, Black Caribbean people living in the UK are disproportionately likely to be diagnosed with schizophrenia, with one seminal study in 2006 finding that we are nine times more likely to receive this diagnosis than our white counterparts.[3] Notably, this extremely high rate of diagnosis in the UK has not been replicated in the Caribbean[4] – suggesting that these rates are more to do with the social and political experiences of Black British people. Since the experiences described as schizophrenia are often thought to be linked to stress and trauma, these rates of diagnosis might be considered entirely representative of our lived realities. I grew up hearing stories of my Antiguan grandmother being invited to board a ship to England, only to be chased down the street by violent white nationalists when she stepped onto its hostile shores. Living in contemporary Britain continues to be traumatising for many people of colour – with racism embedded in each of its institutions.

However, in understanding the disproportionate rate of schizophrenia diagnoses, it is also necessary to interrogate

---

2   R. W. Gilmore, *Golden Gulag: Prisons, Surplus, Crisis, and Opposition in Globalizing California* (Berkeley, CA: University of California Press, 2007).

3   P. Fearon, J. Kirkbride, C. Morgan, et al. 'Incidence of schizophrenia and other psychoses in ethnic minority groups: results from the MRC ÆSOP Study', *Psychol Med*, 36:11, (2006), 1541–50.

4   R. Pinto, M. Ashworth, R. Jones, 'Schizophrenia in black Caribbeans living in the UK: an exploration of underlying causes of the high incidence rate', *Br J Gen Pract*, 58:551(Jun 2008), pp. 429–34.

the racism that is embedded in the foundations of psychiatry. Racism is intimately tied to the history of psychiatric diagnosis; most famously, the American physician Samuel A. Cartwright proposed the diagnosis of 'drapetomania' in 1851 to describe Black enslaved people who fled from plantations.[5] The schizophrenia diagnosis, which originates from a nineteenth century diagnosis called 'dementia praecox', has a similarly racialised history. Psychiatrists influenced by eugenics saw dementia praecox as associated with Black 'degeneracy' and 'primitiveness'.[6] The British colonial psychiatrist H. L. Gordon, who worked in a Kenyan mental hospital in the 1930s, even suggested that African people developed the disorder due to the 'inferior durability' of their brain cells.[7]

After a brief period of its usage as a 'housewife's disease' in the mid-twentieth century, schizophrenia was once again subtly naturalised as a Black illness in the late 1960s.[8] When the second edition of the DSM was released in 1968, the diagnostic criteria described schizophrenia as making people 'hostile' and 'aggressive'[9] – attributes that overlap with stereotypes of Black violence and criminality. During this period, Black people in the US and Britain were increasingly diagnosed with schizophrenia. The systematic diagnosis of schizophrenia among Black people was further used to pathologise their direct and organised responses to systemic racism. In the 1960s, the

---

5   S. Cartwright, *Report on the Diseases and Physical Peculiarities of the Negro Race* (New Orleans: New Orleans Medical and Surgical Journal, 1851).

6   R. J. Barrett, 'Conceptual foundations of schizophrenia: I. Degeneration', *Australian and New Zealand Journal of Psychiatry* 32, (1998), pp. 617–26.

7   S. Mahone and M. Vaughan (eds), *Psychiatry and Empire* (Basingstoke: Palgrave Macmillan UK, 2007).

8   Metzl, *The Protest Psychosis*.

9   American Psychiatric Association, *Dsm-ii: Diagnostic and Statistical Manual of Mental Disorders*, second edition (1968).

US psychiatrists Walter Bromberg and Franck Simon suggested that Malcolm X and the civil rights movement had sparked a wave of violent schizophrenic symptoms and paranoid 'racial antagonism' in Black Americans. As more Black people joined the movement and consciously dissented against the racist societal order, Bromberg and Simon dubbed this phenomenon 'the protest psychosis'.[10] The ongoing association between schizophrenia, violence and criminality undoubtedly still plays a role in the disproportionate number of Black people who are diagnosed. Black men, in particular, who experience mass criminalisation by the state, are now 10 times more likely to receive a diagnosis of a psychotic disorder than their white counterparts.[11]

Racism also factors into how the world *responds* to Black people's genuine mental distress. Since psychiatry has largely located Black people's distress inside of their bodyminds rather than in their environments, Caribbean Britons have historically been disproportionately subject to risky and invasive physical interventions like electroconvulsive therapy (ECT) and major tranquilisers rather than more socially oriented approaches like psychotherapy.[12,13] Most of these issues persist into the present-day, as Black people are still nearly five times as likely to be detained under the Mental Health Act than their white counterparts.[14] They are also more likely to make contact with mental

---

10   Metzl, *The Protest Psychosis*.

11   www.ethnicity-facts-figures.service.gov.uk/health/mental-health/adults-experiencing-a-psychotic-disorder/latest (last accessed January 2023).

12   R. Littlewood and S. Cross, 'Ethnic Minorities and Psychiatric Services', *Sociology of Health & Illness*, 2, (1980), pp. 194–201.

13   S. Scafe, S. Dadzie and B. Bryan, *The Heart of the Race: Black Women's Lives in Britain* (London and New York: Verso Books, 2018).

14   https://ethnicity-facts-figures.service.gov.uk/health/mental-health/detentions-under-the-mental-health-act/latest (last accessed January 2023).

health services through the police and criminal justice system, less likely to gain access to psychological therapies, disproportionately likely to be on a medium or high secure ward, and also more likely to be secluded and restrained on wards.[15] Black distress is interpreted through the psychiatric gaze as irrational, dangerous and primal – something to be dominated rather than understood.

Even in the therapy room, people of colour – who frequently only have access to white therapists – often report facing covert or overt racism. In 2017, I worked with students of colour to compile a report on their experiences in therapy. In a survey of 143 students and alumni, a significant number of people said that white therapists had stereotyped them, adopted culturally inappropriate lines of questioning, or questioned whether their experiences of racism were really 'real'.[16] The most common concern students raised was that they had to spend a large amount of session time simply explaining basic elements of racism or their culture. As we organised around these concerns, other students and I also found ourselves struggling with a therapeutic institution that saw itself as neutral and apolitical. Ultimately, many students found that the only forums equipped to hold their experiences were explicitly political consciousness-raising groups and peer support spaces. We came to learn that, while the therapy room can be a place of support and healing, it can also reproduce racial violence through unequal power dynamics and the desire for individualism and 'objectivity'.

---

15   https://mind.org.uk/news-campaigns/legal-news/legal-newsletter-june-2019/ discrimination-in-mental-health-services/ (last accessed January 2023).

16   https://theguardian.com/commentisfree/2018/may/21/identity-matters-black-students-black-therapists-cambridge-university (last accessed January 2023).

Bordering Madness

Nation states, and the borders that maintain them, work by exclusion. Borders determine who is in and who is out. Many people who are forced to cross borders have experienced conflict and persecution in their home countries and endure life-threatening journeys to make their way to safety. In the countries they migrate to, they are often made into second-class citizens. Migration status can determine who has access to shelter, healthcare, travel, employment and, crucially, who does not. It therefore follows that borders produce Madness and disability; 61% of asylum seekers experience serious mental distress, and refugees are five times more likely to have 'mental health needs' than the rest of the population. Migrants and their children are significantly more likely to meet the criteria for post-traumatic stress disorder (PTSD) – particularly when children are separated from their parents.

In 2012, former UK Home Secretary Theresa May began to introduce policies that to this day attack the wellbeing and human rights of migrants and racialised people. May said at the time: 'The aim is to create, here in Britain, a really hostile environment for illegal immigrants.' 'Hostile environment' policies work to prevent undocumented migrants from accessing services like the NHS, and from being able to legally get a job and rent a home. They also ensure that borders are not only concrete boundaries on the outskirts of nation states, but present throughout society by bringing them into services, communities and homes. Policies require police, doctors, landlords and teachers to act as border guards, asking for proof of migration status if a person appears to be 'foreign'.[17] Leah Cowan,

---

17 https://jcwi.org.uk/the-hostile-environment-explained (last accessed January 2023).

author of *Border Nation*, who also works at an advice centre that supports migrant families, tells me:

> In practice, the hostile environment creates a constant state of fear and precarity, which is going to chip away at your well-being. If we don't have our basic needs met, we can't be well. This is the function of the hostile environment: to make sure you can't rent anywhere to live, you can't get a job, you can't access healthcare. The border does everything in its power to mentally destroy you – I genuinely believe that's the intention.

Britain's immigration detention system, which we touched on in Chapter 1, also produces mass suffering through incarcerating people who are deemed to be 'illegal'. Thousands of people enter immigration detention in the UK each year – with numbers peaking in 2015 at 32,000.[18] The conditions in detention centres mirror those of prisons: cells, bunkbeds, the removal of bodily autonomy, guards, cell lock-ins, and toilets that are in plain sight of others.[19] Detainees are usually given no time limit on how long they will be incarcerated for – Cowan says: 'in prison, you're counting down the days, whereas in immigration detention, you're counting *up*'. Studies unsurprisingly show that people who are detained in immigration detention facilities face anxiety, fear, hopelessness, sleep problems, self-harm and suicidal thoughts.[20] These conditions would be maddening for

---

18 https://gov.uk/government/statistics/immigration-statistics-year-ending-march-2021/how-many-people-are-detained-or-returned (last accessed January 2023).

19 https://theguardian.com/uk-news/2018/oct/11/life-in-a-uk-immigration-removal-centre-worse-than-prison-as-criminal-sentence (last accessed January 2023).

20 https://rcpsych.ac.uk/docs/default-source/improving-care/better-mh-policy/position-statements/position-statement-ps02-21---detention-of-people-with-mental-disorders-in-immigration-removal-centres---2021.pdf (last accessed January 2023).

anyone, but Cowan tells me they can have uniquely devastating mental health impacts for the 27% of detainees in Britain who have previously been victims of torture:[21] 'the sound of jangling keys and locking doors is often really triggering for their PTSD'.

Mental health systems and immigration systems also overlap and collude with one another to serve the interests of the state. As mentioned, under hostile environment policies, doctors are encouraged to enquire about patients' immigration status and share information with the Home Office. Patients who are not 'ordinarily resident' are also charged for accessing services. Cowan tells me:

> Whether you have a pre-existing mental health issue or you've had one induced by your engagement with the border regime, you can't even ask for help with it. People feel disinclined to go and see doctors, therapists, counsellors, charities … support groups, because they're worried about immigration enforcement action being taken.

In countries like the US and Canada, the borders of Mad/sane can be used to bolster the borders of the nation state. For example, people can be barred from entering or gaining a US green card if they are seen to have a 'physical or mental disorder that can be clinically diagnosed', and 'behavior associated with the disorder that could pose or has posed a threat to the property, safety or welfare of the immigrant or to others in the public'.[22] These judgments are subjective, but demonstrate how sanity is tied to the construct of the 'good' and submissive nation state subject, in the interest of protecting capital.

---

21 https://theguardian.com/uk-news/2018/oct/10/revealed-sick-tortured-immigrants-locked-up-for-months-in-britain (last accessed January 2023).
22 https://uscis.gov/policy-manual/volume-8-part-b-chapter-7 (last accessed January 2023).

Intimately tied to the UK's borders is its legacy of colonialism, and the global suffering it has caused. In the 1950s and 1960s, the Martiniquais psychiatrist Frantz Fanon drew links between colonial violence and emotional suffering – arguing against the idea that colonised people were primitive or inferior because of their mental distress. Fanon believed that colonialism had a significant role in shaping the psyche and a person's entire sense of self. The trauma brought about by colonial violence also has knock-on emotional, social and economic effects that ripple across generations and communities and therefore cannot be measured on the level of the individual. Nonetheless, the psychiatric approach to colonial suffering largely treats it as a personal problem. For example, some psychiatrists have recently proposed the diagnostic term 'residential school syndrome' to describe the post-traumatic stress faced by survivors of Canada's residential school system.[23] These institutions, established by settler colonisers in the nineteenth century on Turtle Island,[24] worked to eradicate the culture of indigenous First Nations, Inuit and Métis peoples, and saw children separated from their families, beaten, sexually abused, malnourished, experimented on, neglected and killed by disease. But since medicine and psychiatry largely adopt an individualist approach to suffering, the medical concept of a *syndrome* serves to depoliticise the impacts of colonial violence, as argued by Fanon. Through the Western medical gaze, the focus is shifted to the trauma responses of indigenous people, to be remedied in the clinic rather than through structural or economic reparations.

23 C. R. Brasfield, 'Residential school syndrome', *British Columbia Medical Journal* 43:2, (2001), pp. 78–81.
24 This term is most frequently used by indigenous peoples to refer to North America.

Psychiatric forms of mental health knowledge also colonise others. Cultures across the globe have their own indigenous knowledge systems through which they have long understood Madness/Mental Illness and distress. During colonial expansion, Western individualist medical, psychological and psychiatric understandings were exported across the world. Colonial asylums began to be established at the same time that they were rolled out en masse across Britain – and by the turn of the twentieth century, there were 26 asylums in India alone. Today, medical and psychiatric understandings continue to expand across cultures, with the World Health Organisation (WHO) and a Movement for Global Mental Health calling for psychiatric interventions to be scaled up across the world.[25] I have seen the harms of this kind of psychiatric imperialism in my own community in Britain. In many African and Caribbean cultures, the 'symptoms' associated with schizophrenia diagnoses are not understood as pathological, but rather as having particular spiritual meanings. My mother grew up in the Pentecostal church, in which churchgoers were encouraged to 'get in the spirit', shake, laugh, shout, dance, speak 'in tongues' and communicate with the voice of God. According to the psychiatric standard in Britain, these were signs of schizophrenia, and saw my family members pathologised. The impact of this was the control of racialised people and their various ways of making meaning in the world.

Restricting transness

Being trans in our society, for many, means being subjected to violence in a variety of forms. It may be overt – 41% of trans

---

25   C. Mills, *Decolonizing Global Mental Health: The Psychiatrization of the Majority World* (London: Routledge, 2014).

men and women have experienced a hate crime or incident because of their gender identity.[26] Rejection from family, landlords and employers also means that transphobia has material impacts on living and working conditions. Twenty-five per cent of trans people have been homeless at some point in their lives.[27] Meanwhile 65% say that they feel it is necessary to keep their identity secret from colleagues to feel safe and secure in their jobs.[28] This economic precariousness means that trans people are also more likely to be forced into mentally harmful living and working conditions. Meanwhile, trans people are also systematically denied access to vital healthcare. Over 10,000 trans people sit on a waiting list for gender-affirming medical care in the UK,[29] with the average wait time for an appointment being two years.[30] These conditions have only become worse in recent years, as commentators, politicians and hate groups have systematically whipped up transphobia and have made it harder for trans people to live in peace.

Seventy-seven percent of trans people have had suicidal thoughts or feelings.[31] This is not a biological inevitability, a strange comorbidity or because trans people are simply confused about who they are and what they need. Rather, this is a direct product of trans people's material conditions. My friend Kate, whose sister Alice died by suicide while waiting for gender-affirming care, tells me: 'Alice's feelings of hopelessness are inseparable from the inaccessibility of trans healthcare in the

---

26   https://stonewall.org.uk/lgbt-britain-trans-report (last accessed January 2023).
27   Ibid.
28   https://theguardian.com/society/2021/mar/22/more-trans-people-hiding-identity-at-work-than-five-years-ago-report (last accessed January 2023).
29   https://gic.nhs.uk/appointments/waiting-times/ (last accessed January 2023).
30   https://metro.co.uk/2022/07/23/in-focus-nhs-waiting-times-leaving-trans-people-broke-and-on-the-brink-17019469/ (last accessed January 2023).
31   https://theguardian.com/society/2021/may/17/lgbt-youths-twice-as-likely-to-contemplate-suicide-survey-finds (last accessed January 2023).

UK, and the political project to exclude trans people from public life. The barriers Alice faced to her happiness were material and structural, and cannot be overcome through "raising awareness" or "ending stigma". When Alice died, she had been on the NHS Gender Identity Clinic waiting list for 1,023 days, which Kate says undoubtedly played a role in her suicide. Just a month before her death, she had contacted her GP in Brighton to say that she didn't feel life was worth living. But Kate tells me that broader societal hostility towards trans people also made Alice too frightened to participate in public life. Alice wrote in a poem that her family discovered after her death: 'I can't go out alone, I can't get on a train'.

Historically, psychiatry has categorised trans people as Mad. 'Transvestitism' has appeared in the DSM since its first edition – far predating the current biological paradigm. Trans people, like gay people, were subject to conversion shock therapies on the NHS until the 1970s, demonstrating how psychiatry has long colluded with eugenic desires to control and forcibly change deviant bodyminds.

After being 'depathologised' by the DSM in 2012, and by the International Classification of Diseases (ICD) in 2019, many trans people are still psychiatrised under the diagnosis of gender dysphoria, which appears in the DSM-5.[32] For most trans medical interventions in the UK, a diagnosis of gender dysphoria is necessary to receive state medical support, demonstrating how psychiatry and medicine continue to exercise control over trans bodyminds. In this system, psychiatrists are granted the power to define what constitutes 'real' dysphoria, and can decide which trans people are considered worthy of medical care. Harry Josephine Giles, a writer and performer who has written on anti-psychiatry and transness, tells me:

32   At the time of writing, this is the most recent edition of the DSM.

Trans people [must perform] their transness to psychiatrists' demands, developing plausible narratives of themselves that meet the criteria for diagnosis. In this way, psychiatrists have created the frames through which we understand what transness even is. All this arises from one counterintuitive but evident fact: psychiatry exists not to assist transition, but to limit the number of people who transition and how they transition. Psychiatry creates processes to deny trans healthcare, a tight mesh of restrictive ideas through which gender diverse people are forced to squeeze themselves.

However, if a person has other psychiatric diagnoses on their record, they may also struggle to get a gender dysphoria diagnosis, and be barred from transition. Paradoxically, transness is therefore simultaneously framed as incompatible with Madness, and as a form of Madness in itself. The idea that being trans is a form of Madness/Mental Illness is not only visible in medical settings. Broader transphobic rhetoric in the public sphere still often leans heavily on the idea that trans people are Mad, need curing, and therefore don't deserve the right to bodily autonomy. Therefore societal violence towards trans people cannot be disentangled from violence towards Mad/Mentally Ill people – both are constructed by the state as problems of deviance to be controlled.

Can money buy happiness?

More than one in five people in the UK live in poverty,[33] a group that is disproportionately made up of people of colour, disabled people and women.[34] Nine percent of the world's population lives

---

33   https://jrf.org.uk/data/overall-uk-poverty-rates (last accessed January 2023).
34   https://bigissue.com/news/social-justice/uk-poverty-the-facts-figures-effects-solutions-cost-living-crisis/ (last accessed January 2023).

in extreme poverty,[35] a reality shaped by the ongoing impacts of colonialism. The Socialist Patients' Collective (SPK), the radical German patients' group mentioned in Chapter 1, once wrote that illness is the 'only possible form of life in capitalism.'[36] It makes all of us sick. However, the impossibility of 'mental health' under capitalism is more apparent for people living in poverty.

In the 1940s, the psychologist Abraham Maslow theorised that there was a pyramid-shaped hierarchy of human needs – with physiological necessities like food, water and shelter at the bottom, and then things like self-esteem and self-actualisation towards the top. Maslow felt that a person couldn't fulfil the psychological needs towards the top of the pyramid if they didn't have their basic needs met. While there are clear faults with this kind of 'ranking' system of needs (which are, in actuality, more fluid and intertwined), we must acknowledge that some people become unwell because they are denied access to very basic needs. How can a person *not* be depressed or anxious when they are working multiple jobs to pay their rent? Or when they don't know where they are going to get their next meal from, or if they will have a place to sleep tonight? In these situations, what we describe as depression might also be a clear response to untenable living conditions – anxiety, a response that propels a person forward and keeps them alive. Eighty percent of homeless people in England report having mental health issues.[37]

Being Mad/Mentally Ill also plummets many people into poverty. As we will discuss in more detail in the following

---

35 https://www.worldbank.org/en/topic/poverty/overview (last accessed January 2023).

36 Sozialistisches Patientenkollektiv, *SPK, Turn Illness into a Weapon for Agitation by the Socialist Patients' Collective at the University of Heidelberg*, KRRIM, 1993.

37 WHO, 'Global burden of mental disorders and the need for a comprehensive, coordinated response from health and social sectors at the country level: Report by the Secretariat', 2011.

chapter, the labour market excludes a large proportion of Mad/ Mentally Ill and disabled people by design – because it is harder to extract labour from these bodyminds. This kind of exclusion from employment can trigger a vicious cycle of mental ill health; if you cannot access work because you are too unwell, you are likely to become more distressed because of your situation, and therefore less able to work. This can trigger a phenomenon described by some as 'social drift', a process whereby Mad/ Mentally Ill people slowly drift into poverty, even when they didn't start off there. The cycles continue, with more factors thrown into the mix: if you become homeless, how will you get a job to get out of homelessness? If you are visibly unwell, how can you avoid being sectioned under the Mental Health Act if you don't have a home to go inside?

While liberal awareness-raising narratives suggest that stigma is what stops people from getting adequate support, a large factor, for most people, is money. In 2017, Emily May wrote for *Blueprint* in a piece called *Mental illness is expensive*:[38]

Medication promised quick and cost-effective respite . . . Multiple medical professionals have recommended that I find long-term private psychotherapy . . . Neither shame nor taboo keeps me from going; those ships sailed long ago. It's that I can't afford it.

While richer people can afford more costly therapies that aren't widely available on the NHS (for example, psychotherapy), poorer people invariably get cheaper state solutions like medication and CBT. They also have to weather years-long waiting lists, and are more likely to get to crisis point before they get any

38 https://blueprintzine.com/portfolio/mental-illness-is-expensive-why-austerity-makes-me-sad/ (last accessed January 2023).

'support' for their suffering (which, at this stage, is more likely to come in the form of state detention, compulsory treatment and further traumatisation).

However, capitalism has the potential to erode *all* forms of 'health' and joy – even for those who might consider themselves better off. We all live under a system characterised by dog-eat-dog individualist competition. Some people may be 'winning' at this game. However, almost everyone bears some psychic impact of this system. We can see this in the widespread need to always be 'succeeding' by a narrow capitalist metric; our constant lust for material commodities that we might not even really want or need; the decimation of community; the corruption of our inter-actions with almost all other people into processes of extraction and exchange, rather than care and solidarity; the fact that everyone seems to be 'stressed'; constant, ever-present loneli-ness. The capitalist tenets of extraction, exploitation and greed pose a psychic risk to all of us, and are antithetical to 'health'.

The world is making us Mad

The national and global suffering that we see in the form of mental health statistics cannot be viewed in a political vacuum. The world makes us Mad, and then goes on to define who is pathologised as Mad, and how they are treated. Despite the way that we have approached the issues covered in this chapter – looking at a few select matrices of oppression – this is by no means an exhaustive list. Rather, these are particularly clear examples that speak to the social contours of the mental health crisis. We should also remember that these systems are not really separate at all – they are interlocked, and reinforce one another. Most people are impacted by more than one system. As the feminist Audre Lorde has written, we do not live single-issue lives. We should therefore unite our analysis of each of these systems, in particular, the ways that they are all shaped by capitalism, to understand how to tear them down.

In 1963, Martin Luther King gave a speech at Western Michigan University, in which he advocated for what he called 'maladjustment'. The word is traditionally a psychological label that describes a person's failure to 'healthily' adjust to their social environment, however King wanted to take a more creative and political approach to the term. He said:

> There are certain things in our nation and in the world which I am proud to be maladjusted . . . I never intend to become adjusted to segregation and discrimination ... I never intend to adjust myself to economic conditions that will take necessities from the many to give luxuries to the few, leave millions of God's children smothering in an airtight cage of poverty in the midst of an affluent society. I never intend to adjust myself to the madness of militarism, to self-defeating effects of physical violence.[39]

As King has suggested, to be maladjusted, distressed or Mad – while often deeply distressing – can also be a response to intolerable conditions that a person cannot adjust to. If we wish to see our suffering in this way, then to be Mad, as in 'angry', can be interpreted as a form of protest. It is no coincidence that so many of us come to radical politics through experiences of trauma. Distress is not only a signal or symptom; it can also be a driving force that fuels all of our movements and guides us towards liberation. As King argued: 'Through such maladjustment, I believe that we will be able to emerge from the bleak and desolate midnight of man's inhumanity . . . into the bright and glittering daybreak of freedom and justice.'

---

39   https://youtube.com/watch?v=zXEIYpnlxbw (last accessed January 2023).

Chapter 4

Why work is sickening

The worker [. . .] only feels himself outside his work, and in his work feels outside himself. He feels at home when he is not working, and when he is working he does not feel at home. – Karl Marx

Being human is an absurd and ridiculous career, and sanity is the jobsworth in charge. – Dolly Sen

This chapter contains discussions of suicide.

Since the days of the industrial revolution, the production line has been dangerous. In the eighteenth and nineteenth centuries, as manufacturing processes changed in nature and demand, societies saw a proliferation of new diseases that were particular to conditions of work: lung disease, dermatitis, and 'phossy jaw', the death of cells in the jaw due to phosphorus exposure in the match industry.[1] Images of Victorian Britain are always peppered with images of disability – people who were injured by explosions in coal mines, children who lost limbs or fingers to high-speed and uncontrollable machinery, people disabled by smog and disease in cramped cities organised around the factory.[2] Colonised people, whose enslaved labour funded the

---

1 https://medicalnewstoday.com/articles/323538 (last accessed January 2023).
2 F. Engels and V. G. Kiernan, *The Condition of the Working Class in England* (London: Penguin Books, 1987).

revolution taking place on Britain's mainland, lived their lives in constant proximity to sickness and death, becoming ill, disabled and scarred through inhumane living conditions and brutal punishments.[3]

However, in the mid-nineteenth century, the theorist Karl Marx also began to turn his attention to the psychic and relational injuries that result from the capitalist mode of production, in his theory of 'alienation'.[4] Marx observed that workers were estranged from their work, the things that they produced, from their co-workers and from themselves. Under the capitalist system, workers only produced because they would die if they didn't, and the terms with which they engaged with work were dictated by external forces – the boss, the boss' boss, the board and the markets. Workers therefore became fundamentally dissociated from the capacity for joy and connection, a psychic wound that accompanied each of the physical ones sustained during work. Although the last two centuries have seen conditions of production shift across time and space, it remains true that capitalist work harms our entire bodyminds through exploitation and the quest for profit.

Today, many of the world's most profitable businesses foster working conditions that are health-destroying in the immediate short term. At Amazon, one of the most valuable companies in the world, conditions for their poor and racialised workers resemble the speed and mechanism of the factory line; warehouse workers and drivers are subject to rigorous time-tracking, with a number of workers reporting that they had developed

---

3 S. Hunt-Kennedy, *Between Fitness and Death: Disability and Slavery in the Caribbean* (Urbana: University of Illinois Press, 2020).

4 K. Marx, *Economic and Philosophic Manuscripts of 1844*, trans. M. Milligan (Dover Publications, 2007).

UTIs[5] because they do not have time to go to the toilet at work.[6] Meanwhile, 40% of Amazon employees have experienced pain or injury at work, and of those workers who said they had acquired a serious injury, 80% said it was related to production speed or pressure.[7] In 2021, 159 Apple workers in India were hospitalised with food poisoning, after which it was discovered that they had been forced to live off of worm-infested food, in rat-infested dorms, with no running water.[8]

Many businesses take these health risks with the understanding that when their workers' bodies wear and break, they can be replaced, like any other piece of equipment. Even before the pandemic, Amazon replaced over 150 per cent of its hourly workers every year[9] – meaning that the high number of lifelong injuries sustained at the company are of little consequence to profit margins.[10] Wal-Mart, parent company to Asda and one of the most profitable businesses in the world, follows a similar business model – with at least 3% of workers injured each year,[11] and an annual turnover rate of 70%.[12] The 'gig economy', which has seen a spike in precarious work in recent decades, has only

5   https://theatlantic.com/technology/archive/2019/11/amazon-warehouse-reports-show-worker-injuries/602530/ (last accessed January 2023).

6   https://theatlantic.com/technology/archive/2019/11/amazon-warehouse-reports-show-worker-injuries/602530/ (last accessed January 2023).

7   https://thesoc.org/amazon-primed-for-pain/ (last accessed January 2023).

8   https://reuters.com/world/india/women-force-change-indian-iphone-plant-sick-bad-food-crowded-dorms-2021-12-30/ (last accessed January 2023).

9   https://theguardian.com/technology/2022/jun/22/amazon-workers-shortage-leaked-memo-warehouse (last accessed January 2023).

10   https://marketplace.org/2021/06/18/amazon-workforce-turnover-dominance-investigation/ (last accessed January 2023).

11   https://vice.com/en/article/epnvpn/injury-data-shows-amazon-jobs-are-more-dangerous-than-walmart-and-ups (last accessed January 2023).

12   https://equitablegrowth.org/how-a-large-employers-low-road-practices-harm-local-labor-markets-the-impact-of-walmart-supercenters/ (last accessed January 2023).

allowed this approach to workers' health to further proliferate – with high risk of occupational pain[13] and injury.[14,15] Due to an 'oversupply' of labourers, certain employers aren't motivated to change – they can simply change their workers. Profit ultimately comes over health.

Work's mental toll

As Marx argued, work does not only take its toll in the form of physical injuries, strains and toxins. As the activity that occupies the greatest proportion of our waking hours, it is naturally connected to our emotional and psychic experience of the world. In the year 2020–21, 822,000 British workers reported work-related stress, depression and anxiety.[16] The previous year, 17.9 million working days were lost to these forms of work-related distress, the highest proportion of working days lost to any work-related health concern.[17] Seventy-nine per cent of UK workers report that they have suffered from 'burnout'.[18] Nonetheless, these statistics undoubtedly downplay the true scale of the problem – because we *all* suffer under our current working conditions, in ways that are not always neatly statistically measurable.

13   A. J. Wood, M. Graham, V. Lehdonvirta and I. Hjorth, 'Good Gig, Bad Gig: Autonomy and Algorithmic Control in the Global Gig Economy', *Work, Employment and Society*, 33:1, (2019), pp. 56–75.

14   Y. Morita, K. Kandabashi, S. Kajiki, H. Saito, G. Muto and T. Tabuchi, 'Relationship between occupational injury and gig work experience in Japanese workers during the COVID-19 pandemic: a cross-sectional internet survey', *Industrial Health*, 60:4, (2022), pp. 360–70.

15   https://mirror.co.uk/money/jobs/gig-economy-workers-injured-work-25587129 (last accessed January 2023).

16   https://hse.gov.uk/statistics/causdis/stress.pdf (last accessed January 2023).

17   https://hse.gov.uk/statistics/dayslost.htm (last accessed January 2023).

18   O. C. Tanner, *2019/2020 Global Culture Report*, https://octanner.com/global-culture-report.html (last accessed January 2023).

Precarious work is closely associated with mental distress. Hospitality workers experience the highest reported levels of workplace stress out of any industry;[19,20] and those who rely on tips are at a particularly high risk of depression and sleep problems.[21] These occupational hazards are exacerbated by 'emotional labour'[22] – the process of having to control, mask and split off certain emotions when faced with customer hostility or even sexual harassment – which disproportionately affects women in the service industries. Work alienates and dissociates them from their feelings, which are no longer theirs.[23]

Many of the world's largest and most physically hazardous manufacturers have equally damning track records for worker mental health. At Foxconn's factory in Shenzhen, China, where Apple iPhones are manufactured, 17 workers took their own lives over a five-year period,[24] with a number of other reported suicide attempts.[25] 'It's not a good place for human beings', one former employee told the *Guardian*.[26] During another five-year period in the US, there were at least 189 calls to emergency services regarding 'suicide attempts, suicidal thoughts and

19   https://publicsectorcatering.co.uk/news/hospitality-workers-amongst-most-stressed-britain-research-finds (last accessed January 2023).

20   https://cateringinsight.com/hospitality-industry-named-most-stressful-for-workers/ (last accessed January 2023).

21   S. B. Andrea, L. C. Messer, M. Marino and J. Boone-Heinonen, 'Associations of tipped and untipped service work with poor mental health in a nationally representative cohort of adolescents followed into adulthood', *American Journal of Epidemiology*, 187:10, (October 2018), pp. 2177–85.

22   A. R. Hochschild, *The Managed Heart*, third edition, (Berkeley, Los Angeles and London: University of California Press, 2012).

23   Ibid.

24   https://wired.com/2011/02/ff-joelinchina/ (last accessed January 2023).

25   https://theguardian.com/technology/2017/jun/18/foxconn-life-death-forbidden-city-longhua-suicide-apple-iphone-brian-merchant-one-device-extract (last accessed January 2023).

26   Ibid.

other mental health episodes' from Amazon warehouses.[27] Jace Crouch, an employee who had an emotional crisis on the job, told the *Daily Beast*: '[it's] mentally taxing to do the same task super fast for 10-hour shifts, four or five days a week',[28] also saying that employee breakdowns were a regular occurrence.

While suicide is a clear manifestation of the impacts of mental suffering on the physical body; in other cases, stress may become more quietly inscribed on the body in the form of physical illness. Musculoskeletal disorders (from tensing) and cardiovascular disease have been consistently linked to work-related stress;[29,30] meanwhile stress has also been linked to fatigue, gastrointestinal problems, the immune system, the reproductive system and a host of other bodily functions.[31] One analysis by the business theorist Jeffrey Pfeffer found that work stress was the fifth leading cause of death in the US, above alzheimer's and kidney disease.[32] Therefore work-related mental and physical suffering can become a vicious circle, with each fuelling the other.

Lower ranks, higher stress

Most workplaces are hierarchical, and long-term research has shown that mental and physical health impacts of work cluster

27   https://thedailybeast.com/amazon-the-shocking-911-calls-from-inside-its-warehouses (last accessed January 2023).

28   Ibid.

29   M. Kivimäki and I. Kawachi, 'Work stress as a risk factor for cardiovascular disease', *Curr Cardiol Rep*, 17(9):630, (Sep 2015).

30   G. A. Ariëns, W. van Mechelen, P. M. Bongers, L. M. Bouter and G. van der Wal, 'Psychosocial risk factors for neck pain: a systematic review', *American Journal of Industrial Medicine*, 39:2, (2001), pp. 180–93.

31   https://apa.org/topics/stress/body (last accessed January 2023).

32   J. Pfeffer, *Dying for a Paycheck* (New York: HarperBusiness, 2018).

at the bottom of the ladder. This applies to desk workers as much as it does for those on their feet or on the factory line. The 'Whitehall Studies', an ongoing piece of research that has assessed the health of British civil servants since the 1960s, have found that the lower a person's grade in the civil service, the shorter their predicted lifespan and the more likely they are to die of illnesses like coronary heart disease.[33] Work makes us sick, but it is low-paid, low-ranking work that makes us the sickest. Marx's theory of alienation – which also critiqued the lack of autonomy afforded to workers under capitalism – can further enhance our understanding of the finer detail of these studies. For example, workers who were controlled more closely by their managers took more sick days, and had higher instances of reported Mental Illness, heart disease and pain in the lower back. Marx also argued that workers become alienated from one another as a result of being placed in forcible competition with their co-workers. This is as relevant as ever to the fiercely competitive working environment for low paid gig economy workers in Britain – 7 million of which could lose their jobs at short or no notice.[34]

The mental and physical health impacts found in lower-ranking, lower-paid and precarious job roles are undoubtedly reflective of the labour burden placed on people in these positions; they are usually expected to perform the most strenuous, skilled work, often in hostile, dangerous and competitive working conditions. But we should also think about the knock-on effects of this outside of work, for example, those low-paid workers who

33   M. G. Marmot, G. Rose, M. Shipley and P. J. Hamilton, 'Employment grade and coronary heart disease in British civil servants', *Journal of Epidemiology and Community Health*, 32:4, (Dec 1978), pp. 244–9.
34   https://theguardian.com/uk-news/2016/nov/15/more-than-7m-britons-in-precarious-employment (last accessed January 2023).

must take on multiple jobs to make ends meet, therefore multiplying their work stress. Work-induced distress also speaks to the terrifying realities that work exists in *opposition to*: potential unemployment, poverty, homelessness, and management by the welfare state. The benefits system, which oversees the economic lives of unemployed members of the 'surplus' class,[35,36] can, notably, serve as a death sentence. Therefore the mental burden of work is not limited to a person's shift, and does not end when we clock out. It continues on and on, stretching forward in the imagination into sleepless nights, what-ifs and other forms of anxiety. For many of us, it can feel as if the only way we can possibly ward off these nightmarish outcomes is by working harder, faster, accepting worse terms and conditions, and accepting alienation.

Half a century ago, the radical patient group, the Socialist Patients' Collective (SPK), argued that the process of capitalist production was fundamentally destructive – that it transformed living work into dead matter, and that the proliferation of illness under capitalism was an expression of the same process.[37] Today, our bodyminds remain collateral damage to the process of capitalist production. They may wear, break, or even die. However, this is only significant to the extent that it impacts profit margins. As Marx argued, under this system, workers are reduced to machines with no internal aspiration, fulfilment or agency. If you are able to easily replace your workforce, the profit motive provides no clear rationale to do anything different; employers can keep exploiting our bodyminds until they

35   K. Marx and F. Engels, *Capital. Volume One: A Critique of Political Economy*, trans. B. Fowkes (London: Penguin in association with New Left Review, 1990).

36   B. Adler-Bolton and A. Vierkant, *Health Communism*, (London and New York: Verso, 2022).

37   Sozialistisches Patientenkollektiv, *SPK – Turn Illness into a Weapon for Agitation*.

cannot be exploited any further. Then we are left to pick up the pieces – to find our own way back to 'health'.

Health for exploitation

It would be an oversimplification to say that intentional worker sickness, burnout and mental distress is the *only* reality in workplaces today. While poor health is factored into business models in which workers are viewed as highly replaceable, in other circumstances, it is more cost-effective to remedy worker stress and illness. As a result, in recent centuries, scientists, governments and employers have shown a growing interest in maintaining human bodyminds like any other exploitable resource.

The field of Human Resources can be traced back to at least the nineteenth century. During this period, the American mechanical engineer Fred W. Taylor developed a cluster of principles he called 'scientific management', which aimed to make factory work as empirical, fast and efficient as possible.[38] He conducted experiments where he stood with a stopwatch, just like a modern-day Amazon time-tracker, and analysed workers' motions, looking to fine-tune their bodyminds for better exploitation. In Britain, the field of Human Resources grew and formalised in the twentieth century, during which the Rowntrees and the Cadburys, two families of philanthropic Quakers, began to implement benefits and welfare officers at their factory sites. The government then became concerned about worker welfare during the First World War, as artillery workers became increasingly fatigued, sick and unproductive while manufacturing

---

38   F. W. Taylor, *The Principles of Scientific Management* (New York and London: Harper & Brothers, 1911).

unprecedented amounts of ammunition.[39] Various similar state initiatives followed, investigating the fine details of productivity: the optimum working hours, ventilation, lighting, rest breaks, or workplace layouts that might prevent burnout, and therefore boost productivity.[40]

It is predictable that, over the course of the twentieth century, Human Resources would increasingly orient itself towards the field of psychology, which was gradually gaining power and credibility. The 'Hawthorne Studies', a series of experiments conducted in the 1920s and 1930s, suggested that workers were more productive when they had greater autonomy, social cohesion, people-centred management and feelings of worth – factors that could all be controlled to some extent by employers. By the mid-twentieth century, employers also began to introduce psychometric tests as a part of their hiring practices. There was a clear awareness that workers' emotions and minds needed to be carefully aligned for efficient exploitation, as well as their physical bodies.

Today, 1 in 10 sick days are taken as a result of mental health, and many jobs make not only physical demands, but highly specific cognitive, interpersonal and emotional ones. Despite often destroying our mental well-being, capitalist work (quite paradoxically) has also never been so reliant on us being mentally 'well'. Therefore, while some employers treat workers as entirely disposable, corporate workplaces, in particular, increasingly invest in maintaining workers' bodyminds. This takes the form of benefits like health insurance, but also a growing number of workplace initiatives like free therapy, mindfulness, nap rooms,

---

39 P. N. Rose and N. S. Rose, *Governing the Soul: The Shaping of the Private Self* (London: Routledge, 1990).
40 Ibid.

massages, mental health absence days, wellness and resilience workshops, staff retreats and Mental Health First Aid training.

Focused on aligning our bodyminds with the demands of the market, these techniques serve to simultaneously obscure and legitimise the political and economic forces that lead us to suffer in the first place. Mindfulness is no substitute for a unionised workplace. Nap rooms don't prevent us from working overtime – rather, they help us to do so. Free therapy may make a round of layoffs less psychologically agonising, but it does not prevent them from happening. Individualised workplace mental health initiatives can help us weather the ravages of capitalism with a smile, but they cannot address the root causes of work-related anguish. They do not even begin to touch on the underlying principle that each person must work for a wage to survive; a 'fact of life' that normalises mass death and alienates us from its horror. Workplace mental health interventions also have no internal politics[41] – therapy may help the worker manage their emotions around being fired, or it can help calm the conscience of the boss who is doing the firing. Given this ability to boost productivity[42] and smooth over the emotions associated with exploitative practices, it is no wonder that mindfulness, for example, was imported to the US workplace by Apple CEO Steve Jobs;[43] and continues to be favoured by union-busting CEOs, for both themselves *and* their employees.

In 2010, after the spate of suicides at Foxconn's Shenzhen factory, the manufacturer offered employees counselling as a

---

41   https://theguardian.com/lifeandstyle/2019/jun/14/the-mindfulness-conspiracy-capitalist-spirituality (last accessed January 2023).

42   https://hrmagazine.co.uk/content/features/how-mindfulness-can-improve-productivity (last accessed January 2023).

43   https://news.com.au/technology/innovation/apple-founder-steve-jobs-used-zen-mindfulness-as-path-to-success/news-story/d69f4e281ceabe1e5ae756e833d123b6 (last accessed January 2023).

'solution' to inhumane working conditions, as well as erecting 'anti-suicide nets' below the roof of the building to prevent further deaths.[44] In 2021, after years of bad press, Amazon introduced new mental health benefits for all US employees.[45] These examples are disparate and extreme, but still speak to the overarching capitalist ethos that workers' suffering is an inevitability, and one that can only be remedied on an individual, retrospective basis through the lens of 'mental health support'. Employers keep our bodyminds healthy and well to allow better exploitation within the very system that is harming us. All the while, they create an impression that profit has a moral compass, that it cares about us.

Work constructs 'health'

Work is not only destructive to our mental health. We should also go further to think about how our very notion of 'mental health' is *constructed* in relation to capitalist work. Historically, changes to the conditions of production have ushered in changes in society's understanding of Madness, illness and disability. As we discussed in Chapter 1, the industrial revolution and the emergence of capitalism saw a societal shift from slower, autonomous work in the home to fast-paced, disciplined factory work. This process excluded many people who had previously either been able to participate in the production process, or be cared for in the home.[46]

---

44   https://theguardian.com/technology/2017/jun/18/foxconn-life-death-forbidden-city-longhua-suicide-apple-iphone-brian-merchant-one-device-extract (last accessed January 2023).

45   https://press.aboutamazon.com/2021/5/amazon-introduces-new-mental-health-benefit-for-all-u-s-employees-and-their-family-members (last accessed January 2023).

46   M. Oliver, 'The politics of disablement — new social movements', *The Politics of Disablement: Critical Texts in Social Work and the Welfare State* (London: Palgrave, 1990).

Disability scholars have argued that d/Deaf people, for example, often learned agricultural skills via observation prior to the formal school system, and blind and visually impaired people had greater autonomy and safety in the familiar home environment.[47] The narrow, brutal and alienated working conditions introduced during the industrial revolution, however, pushed sick, Mad and disabled people to the bottom of the market, establishing a class of unemployable people.[48] Their lack of productivity became a problem to be remedied by institutions like prisons, asylums, workhouses, hospitals and schools.[49] Engagement with institutions sorted those who didn't serve the interests of capital into categories like criminal, pauper, disabled, Mad or ill.

As extensions of the capitalist state, the line that these institutions draw between normal and abnormal, productive and unproductive, has always shifted in line with the conditions of production. Throughout history, we have seen a number of changes in who is designated as mentally 'deviant' that support this idea. In the dangerous factory conditions of the 1920s, medical and psychological researchers began to look into the pathology of 'accident-proneness'[50] – an 'affliction' that framed the worker as responsible for their injuries, rather than the factory. Dyslexia, a diagnosis I have been given, also started to be widely recognised and regulated in the twentieth century, as the middle classes emerged and the market began to shift away from manual labour.[51] These changes meant that age-graded schooling

47 E. Topliss, *Provision for the Disabled*, second edition (Oxford: Blackwell with Martin Robertson, 1979).

48 P. Morris, *Put Away* (London: Routledge and Kegan Paul, 1969).

49 Oliver, 'The politics of disablement — new social movements'.

50 M. Greenwood and H. M. Woods, *The Incidence of Industrial Accidents Upon Individuals with Special Reference to Multiple Accidents* (London: H.M. Stationery Off. Darling and Son Ltd., 1919).

51 K. White, *An Introduction to the Sociology of Health and Illness* (London: SAGE Publications Ltd, 2002).

became a compulsory requirement to enter the job market, and children were expected to acquire particular skills at a stand-ardised rate.[52] It is only within this context that a child's reading ability could be diagnosed as falling out of line with the social order, or 'disordered'. My dyslexia was not diagnosed on the basis of my spelling or my ability to recognise words, but because my reading speed is 'too slow'. 'Too slow' for what? Could I be dyslexic in a world without the classroom or the clock? ADHD diagnoses have followed a similar trajectory as work and educa-tion have made greater demands on our attention.[53]

Liberal conversations about Madness/Mental Illness often accept it as a universal, internal, natural fact, but the category has been similarly shaped in relation to capitalist work. Under capitalism, being able to sell our labour is the *definition* of mental health, with 'work' being referenced almost 400 times in the DSM-5.[54] As a result, the common denominator between almost all experiences categorised as Mental Illness is that they, in some way or another, diminish our productivity in work or education (or are otherwise disruptive to the social order in capitalist society). This is reflected in employment statistics – Madness/Mental Illness is the most common reason for benefits claims, at almost 50%.[55] While suffering is often a *component* of Madness/Mental Illness, it is not a precursor. Even when people with particular mental experiences are not actually in distress – for example, someone who hears voices and sees it as a spiritual

52   Ibid.

53   For a materialist analysis of the autism diagnosis, see the work of autistic philosopher Robert Chapman: https://anticapitalistresistance.org/towards-neurodivergent-marxism (last accessed January 2023).

54   Cohen, *Psychiatric Hegemony*.

55   S. Viola and J. Moncrieff, 'Claims for sickness and disability benefits owing to mental disorders in the UK: trends from 1995 to 2014', *British Journal of Psychiatry*, Open:2, (2016), pp. 18–24.

experience – their bodymind may still be categorised as 'ill', because these experiences often limit a person's ability to labour under capitalism. Simultaneously, not all suffering is recognised as Mental Illness; those of us who suffer but are considered 'high functioning' and productive often struggle to have our difficulties medically recognised.[56] While there are so many complex political dimensions to diagnosis, which we will explore in Chapter 6, it is crucial that we understand that our very notion of Madness/Mental Illness is connected to the material conditions of our society. These categories invariably link back to the interests of capital – and who is seen as a contributor to, or a drain on, the economy.

Back to the picket

Our deteriorating mental and physical health is an economic and political problem that requires economic and political solutions. As discussed in Chapter 2, stress and illness have been gradually privatised as a concept since at least the 1980s. Under the current psychiatric paradigm, we largely see suffering as something that takes place within our own bodyminds – when, in actuality, current levels of distress have emerged under the pressures of neoliberal capitalism. The journalist Tim Adams describes this change in focus as a shift 'from picket lines to worry lines'.[57] While it is important to consider the very personal impacts of capitalist work on our bodyminds, we ultimately should not allow this to blunt our political instincts. We all find

56   https://blueprintzine.com/2017/04/21/am-i-sick-enough-on-overlooked-high-functioning-mental-health-problems/ (last accessed January 2023).
57   https://theguardian.com/society/2016/feb/14/workplace-stress-hans-selye (last accessed January 2023).

our ways to psychologically manage the current system, but we also ultimately need to resist it.

It is crucial, then, that we organise with other workers, as well as those excluded and disabled by work. Those in the latter group have attempted to resist mental health initiatives that only serve the purposes of profit. For example, in 2016, the Mental Health Resistance Network called a demonstration in Streatham, South London, to resist the introduction of cognitive behavioural therapy (CBT) in their local Jobcentre. They described it as 'compulsory treatment'[58] with the goal of forcing Mad/Mentally Ill people back into work. In an open letter, they wrote: 'We should not be put under pressure to look for work unless we feel capable. The competitive, profit-driven and exploitative nature of the modern workplace is not suitable for people whose mental health is fragile.'[59] The British service user collective, Recovery in the Bin, has resisted the concept of 'recovery' on similar grounds, writing: 'Capitalism is at the root of the crisis! Many of us will never be able to 'recover' living under these intolerable social and economic conditions.'[60] Workers, who have increasingly organised around health and safety in light of the Covid-19 pandemic, have also shown us that we can take back health for ourselves. In 2022, outsourced cleaners at the private London Bridge Hospital successfully demonstrated and campaigned against poverty pay, lack of sick leave and lack of Covid protections at work.[61,62] These forms of resistance are rehearsals

---

58   https://dpac.uk.net/2015/06/stop-forced-treatments-26th-june-1-30-streatham/ (last accessed January 2023).

59   Ibid.

60   https://recoveryinthebin.org/ritbkeyprinciples/ (last accessed January 2023).

61   https://iwgb.org.uk/en/post/london-bridge-hospital/ (last accessed January 2023).

62   https://independent.co.uk/news/business/hospital-cleaners-covid-ppe-safety-b2014576.html (last accessed January 2023).

for the future we would like to see: one in which workers and non-workers alike have autonomy over our health, and are able to define what 'health' actually looks like.

Liberation for Mad/Mentally Ill people, and all disabled people, demands an end to capitalist work, which, in some way or another, harms, alienates and excludes us all. We internalise work's physical and psychic harms to an extent that we hardly question them at all. But it is worth asking ourselves: to what degree do we value our bodyminds according to their ability to produce for profit? How else could labour be organised to ensure that work did not dictate who is considered worthy or defective, who lives and who dies? Through a shift towards communal labour, living and wealth distribution, we could lay the foundations to finally disentangle illness from work. We might labour because we wanted to, because we loved one another or because not everyone can. We could create conditions that were self-directed, and conducive to life, joy, safety and connection, rather than suffering and destruction. This could apply to all those who laboured, as well as those who didn't. As Marx famously wrote: 'from each according to his [dis]ability, to each according to his needs'.[63]

---

63   K. Marx, *Critique of the Gotha Program*. (n.p.: Wildside Press, 2008).

Chapter 5

Disability/possibility

Disability and Madness is not just an endpoint, but for some, it's also an entry into another site of struggle. – Liat Ben-Moshe

I am dreaming the biggest disabled dream of my life . . . we will leave no one behind as we roll, limp, stim, sign, and move in a million ways towards cocreating the decolonial living future. I am dreaming like my life depends on it. Because it does. – Leah Lakshmi Piepzna-Samarasinha

When I first left my GP's office with a diagnosis of depression and anxiety, I would have never thought of myself as a disabled person. In fact, I suspect that the notion would have seemed ludicrous or even offensive; I had an image of what disability was, and I was not that. Much of my understanding of the concept had likely been shaped by my childhood – I had spent the weekends going with my mum to look after my grandmother, who was blind, had had multiple strokes, was an amputee, and had very limited mobility. As a result, when I thought of disability, I think I would have thought of someone who had mobility aids, full-time care, and physical, permanent barriers to leaving bed or the house. While this is the case for many, I had no idea that at least 70% of disability is considered to be 'invisible'.[1,2]

Disability is rarely afforded depth, breadth or richness as a human experience. In the media, disabled people scarcely seem to exist, except to serve the interests of non-disabled characters and non-disabled audiences. They manifest as moral lessons, strange curiosities, morbid monstrosities, objects of sympathy, or noble artistic challenges that might win actors an Oscar. Off-screen, disability is largely understood as something abject – a thing *not to be*. It is a thing we are told to avoid becoming all our lives, and we are supposed to be grateful if we are *not it*. Even the word 'disabled' is often seen as a sort of slur, or at least a serious allegation, conjuring up words like 'broken' or 'lacking'. It is seen as a shutting down of possibility and opportunity. When people turn over the idea that they might be disabled for the first time, it's not uncommon to have a knee jerk reaction, which says: 'I'm not disabled – there's nothing wrong with me!' But of course, the implication here is that there is something irredeemable about disability.

That day that I got my diagnoses, aged 20, I was at a point in my life where I had already started to untangle concepts like racism, sexism and homophobia; but these ideas about disability remained mostly untouched. In fact, it wasn't until I started to study the politics of mental health in depth that I started to think about the role of disability in my own life, and in my mental health. Looking back, I realise that this was a reflection of the student politics that surrounded me. Disability justice had not been popularised or even co-opted in the way that feminism,

---

1   https://invisibledisabilities.org/what-is-an-invisible-disability/ (last accessed January 2023).

2   https://post.parliament.uk/approved-work-invisible-disabilities/ (last accessed January 2023).

in particular, had been. Few of my friends had become politicised after learning about the disabled people's movement in history lessons, seeing disability justice slogans printed on t-shirts, or having seen Hollywood films about the disabled people's struggle.

This problem persists on the British left more broadly: disability is often framed as something fragmentary, obscure and issue-based, rather than fundamental to broader anti-capitalist thought. Individual diagnostic categories are discussed more than disabled movements. Shrouded in the sterile objectivity and privacy of the institution of medicine, disability is understood as something peripheral and unintelligible that happens 'over there', rather than here in our communities. At political discussions, meetings and organised events, disabled people and their access requirements are treated as hypotheticals – people might talk about what measures they would implement 'if' a disabled person was in the room, forgetting that there is almost *always* a disabled person in said room, whether the organiser realises or not. When groups engage in political actions, accessibility is often either an afterthought, or seen as a financial and logistical hindrance. I have had to leave protests because friends couldn't keep up with the pace of the crowd – left events because organisers cancelled a scheduled break. The exclusion of disabled people from political life even extends to our imaginations; the solitary freedom fighter in the activist's mind is able-bodied, sane and physically strong,[3] as are the people who occupy images of utopia.

This is a relational problem, tarnishing so many disabled people's experiences of political spaces. But it is also a problem of

---

3   D. Goodley, R. Lawthom, K. Liddiard and K. Runswick Cole, 'Critical disability studies', (ed.) Brendan Gough, *The Palgrave Handbook of Critical Social Psychology* (London: Palgrave Macmillan UK, 2017), pp. 491–505.

political education. There is so much that we can all learn from disabled thinking, dreaming and organising, and yet these contributions are usually overlooked. Even in writing this chapter, I have grappled with ways to articulate disability that would stop readers from skimming or flicking ahead to something more interesting. Understanding the transformative power that the politics of disability has had in my own life, I feel defensive in my attempt to convey it as something that is urgent and relevant to mental health, and to all of us.

Disability is an all-encompassing concern. What happens to disabled people means something for us all, in the same way that the demands of other liberation movements – from trans liberation, to labour movements, to the anti-imperialist struggle – affect everyone. At their most radical, these movements do not aim to improve life for 'minorities'. They want to upend the majority, to overthrow systems by grasping them at the root. Therefore 'disabled' isn't just something you are or you are not – it presents us with new ways of understanding the world, and new ways of trying to transform it.

The social model of disability

The current dominant way of thinking about disability draws on the 'medical model'. This model operates on the key idea that disability is a problem located inside the body, which needs to be fixed, usually through engaging with the institution of medicine. But in the 1970s, the Union of the Physically Impaired Against Segregation (UPIAS) – a radical group of physically disabled, London-based Marxists[4] – tried to articulate a new way of thinking about disability. They wrote:

---

4   R. Chapman, *Empire of Normal*.

In our view, it is society which disables physically impaired people. Disability is something imposed on top of our impairments, by the way we are unnecessarily isolated and excluded from full participation in society. Disabled people are therefore an oppressed group in society. It follows from this analysis that having low incomes, for example, is only one aspect of our oppression. It is a consequence of our isolation and segregation, in every area of life, such as education, work, mobility, housing, etc.[5]

This formed the basis for the 'social model', which sees disablement as a force that comes from society, rather than a personal bodily failure. People have impairments, UPIAS argued, but they were *disabled by* their oppressive social environments. The textbook illustration of the social model is the image of a wheelchair user coming up against a flight of stairs at the entrance of a building. While the medical model would say that the problem is that the person cannot walk up stairs, the social model would dictate that the problem is that the building *has stairs*: there is a manmade architectural barrier to the participation of the disabled person.

This rendering of disability has since picked up incredible popularity in both scholarly and activist disability communities. It is explicitly political because it turns the image of disability as a natural fact on its head – drawing attention to the societal forces that oppress disabled people. A social model lens would suggest that disabled people aren't excluded from education and capitalist work because their bodies prevent them from attending, but because these systems are designed to their exclusion. It is education and work that are *disabling*. This shift in emphasis,

---

5   Union of the Physically Impaired Against Segregation (UPIAS), *Fundamental Principles of Disability* (London: UPIAS, 1976).

from blame to barriers, has historically empowered activists to focus on removing social obstacles facing disabled people. In 1995, disabled people launched themselves out of their wheelchairs and onto the floors of train carriages at Cardiff Queen Street station, in protest of inaccessible transport.[6] Others staged protests outside the filming of ITV's *Telethon*, a televised fundraiser for disability charities. Donning T-shirts with the slogan 'PISS ON PITY' emblazoned in bright pink, demonstrators said they wanted rights, not charity.[7] The disabled people's movement in the UK has found power in targeting structures of oppression, resisting the idea that there is anything tragic or inevitable about disabled people's struggles.

The social model also shows how people who experience Madness/Mental Illness or distress can undoubtedly be considered disabled. Just like people who are physically disabled, we are routinely barred from work; with 70% of people in the UK classified as having 'mental illness, phobias, panics or other nervous disorders' being unemployed (excluding depression and anxiety, which is around 50 per cent).[8] Just as physically disabled children have been historically segregated in the school system, half of children expelled from school are reported to have a mental health problem.[9] As I became more involved in disability justice work at university, it also became increasingly obvious to me that I had been battling the same inaccessible education system as my physically disabled peers; trying and

6   https://bbc.co.uk/news/extra/8rvpt6bclh/wheelchair-warriors-disability-discrimination-act (last accessed January 2023).

7   https://medium.com/@theNDACA/block-telethon-1992-the-day-we-pissed-on-pity-69117b03825a (last accessed January 2023).

8   https://researchbriefings.files.parliament.uk/documents/CBP-7540/CBP-7540.pdf (last accessed January 2023).

9   https://theguardian.com/society/2017/jul/20/half-pupils-expelled-school-mental-health-issue-study-finds (last accessed January 2023).

struggling to get lecture notes and extended deadlines. As discussed in Chapter 1, people seen as Mad/Mentally Ill have been institutionalised in a similar way to physically disabled people. These disabling forces concern all of us, even though mental differences might feel less visible than 'physical' disability.

Some disabled people have, however, critiqued the social model's applicability across different disabilities. The UPIAS was a group primarily comprised of wheelchair users, and the model they created is not able to articulate each and every experience of disability. Their focus on removing disabling *barriers* – for example, stairs – has felt incomplete for disabled people who consider their struggles to still have a clear 'medical' or 'internal' component. People who experience chronic illness, pain and fatigue, in particular, have often said that elements of their conditions are inherently disabling, and would be in any society. Alison Kafer argues:

> Social and structural changes will do little to make one's joints stop aching or to alleviate back pain. Nor will changes in architecture and attitude heal diabetes or cancer or fatigue. Focusing exclusively on disabling barriers, as a strict social model seems to do, renders pain and fatigue irrelevant to the project of disability politics.[10]

When I have talked about the social model with other Mad/Mentally Ill people, they have raised similar concerns about its applicability to depression and anxiety. When a person is depressed, they may undoubtedly benefit from things like better sick leave and extended deadlines, but ultimately, may still be suffering on a very fundamental and internal level. No

---

10   Kafer, *Feminist, Queer, Crip.*

amount of barrier removal can change this. Another critique of the model is the artificial binary it erects between impairment and disability. Take the example above – if one feels inherently disabled by low mood or depression, is this an 'impairment' or a 'disability'? And if disability is socially constructed, does that mean that impairment is a natural fact that doesn't also interact with the social world?

In the academic field of disability studies, debates about the social model have raged on for decades, with little clear resolution. Rather than becoming too preoccupied with whether the social model of disability accurately 'explains' disability, it may be more useful to think of it as an imperfect tool. Its historical utility as a political lens is undeniable. But it also has clear limits, and was by no means ever intended to actually be a comprehensive theory of disability. Since its birth, many argue it has been stripped of its radical roots, and lots of other models have been proposed as alternatives, for example, the 'radical model',[11] the 'political/relational model'[12] and the 'money model'.[13,14] Regardless of its shortcomings, the social model can serve as a useful springboard for understanding and a vehicle for radicalisation, showing us that disability does not exist in a political vacuum.

Neurodiversity

'Neurodiversity' has become a buzzword in recent years. More and more people in public life are claiming 'neurodivergence' as

11   A. J. Withers, *Disability Politics and Theory* (Winnipeg, Manitoba: Fernwood Publishing, 2012).

12   Kafer, *Feminist, Queer, Crip*.

13   K. Rosenthal, *Capitalism & Disability: Selected Writings by Marta Russell* (Chicago, Illinois: Haymarket Books, 2019).

14   https://blindarchive.substack.com/p/marta-russell-money-model-of-disability (last accessed January 2023).

a source of personal pride. In the corporate world, conversations circle around the idea that this mysterious ingredient might be a 'competitive advantage',[15] or even a 'superpower'.[16] There is also a growing number of gigs for diversity and inclusion consultants to educate workforces on the importance of neurodiversity awareness in the workplace.[17] But, despite the fact that the term is often colloquially used as an umbrella for diagnoses like autism, ADHD, dyslexia and dyspraxia, 'neurodiversity' is not just a word for people diagnosed with different cognitive or neurological disabilities. Rather, it describes the infinite *neurological diversity* that can be found across humans.[18] The term also has explicit political origins and uses, which have implications for how we might think about mental health.

When autistic people began to connect with each other in the early days of the internet, they challenged the idea that there was something inherently defective in the way they communicated and moved through the world.[19] Subverting the concept of the 'normal' mind or brain, they bemoaned and dissected the strange behaviours of people they described as 'neurologically typical' (or 'neurotypical').[20] When Judy Singer, an autistic Australian sociologist, observed the conversations and philosophies that were developing in this emerging online community, she called, in her 1998 thesis, for a 'politics of neurological diver-

15   https://hbr.org/2017/05/neurodiversity-as-a-competitive-advantage (last accessed January 2023).

16   https://kornferry.com/content/dam/kornferry-v2/pdf/institute/kfi-neurodiversity-the-little-known-superpower.pdf (last accessed January 2023).

17   Chapman, *Empire of Normal*.

18   https://neuroqueer.com/neurodiversity-terms-and-definitions/ (last accessed January 2023).

19   Ibid.

20   https://theatlantic.com/magazine/archive/1998/09/neurodiversity/305909/ (last accessed January 2023).

sity, or neurodiversity', which she saw as the next potential civil rights struggle. The journalist Harvey Blume, who had been in conversation with Singer, described the concept in an article in the *Atlantic* the same year, writing: 'Neurodiversity may be every bit as crucial for the human race as biodiversity is for life in general. Who can say what form of wiring will prove best at any given moment?'[21] Blume's suggestion here was significant – that our conception of 'normal' is socially, culturally and historically bound, and that what is considered 'disordered' in one context might be seen as superior in another.

The autistic author and educator Nick Walker saw these ideas as such a radical break from dominant ways of thinking that she has described them as a 'paradigm shift'[22] – a tearing up of the rulebook that requires rethinking all of our most fundamental assumptions about a topic. Walker considers the old paradigm the 'pathology paradigm', and the new one, the 'neurodiversity paradigm'. While the pathology paradigm suggests that any deviation from the 'norm' is a disorder, the neurodiversity paradigm suggests that neurodiversity is a natural and valuable form of human diversity, and that there is no 'normal' or 'healthy' type of brain or mind.[23] Here, we can see echoes of the social model, in the suggestion that disability is constructed by social forces, rather than being an inherent biological fact.

The neurodiversity paradigm has continued to play a significant role in the politics of autistic communities, in particular. In a similar vein to the online forums of the 1990s, there are large networks of autistic people who find connection and soli-

---

21   Ibid.

22   https://neuroqueer.com/throw-away-the-masters-tools/ (last accessed January 2023).

23   https://neuroqueer.com/neurodiversity-terms-and-definitions/ (last accessed January 2023).

darity on social media, discussing the inaccessibility of the social world, and the strange social conventions of 'neurotypicals'. These communities also promote acceptance, protesting organisations that promote the idea of 'treating', 'curing' or eradicating autistic people in favour of an arbitrary neurotypical norm.[24] These ideas have had a more limited take-up in ADHD communities; however you can find them in pockets. The writer Jesse Meadows has said of their ADHD:

> I don't consider myself a thing to be fixed, but rather, a person who is devalued, disenfranchised, and pushed to assimilate. I don't want to change the socially deviant parts of myself – the parts that make me who I am – I want to change society to accept and accommodate me, along with other disabled and stigmatized people who have it even worse.[25]

Historically, Mad/Mentally Ill activism and neurodiversity activism have sprung from different places, and followed quite separate paths. Today, there is also sometimes an absence of connection between these struggles. For example, the traditional anti-psychiatry movement and its 'critical psychiatry' offshoots generally have not addressed the oppression of people with intellectual and developmental disabilities (I/DD). Equally, the neurodiversity movement has, at times, tried to distance itself from the pathology associated with Mental Illness. But I see Madness/Mental Illness as being included under the umbrella of 'neurodivergent' (a term coined by Kassiane Asasumasu to mean a person who deviates from what is considered the 'normal'

---

24 https://autistichoya.com/2012/11/protesting-autism-speaks.html (last accessed January 2023).

25 https://jessemeadows.medium.com/we-need-critical-adhd-studies-now-52d4267edd54 (last accessed January 2023).

mind or brain). The asylums of the nineteenth century didn't only lock up Mad people, they also incarcerated what we would now call learning disabled and autistic people, who were, at the time, dubbed 'feeble-minded', 'morally defective' or simply Mad. This shared history can be clearly traced to the present day. In 2021, there were 2,075 autistic people and people with learning disabilities in inpatient mental health hospitals, the majority of which were detained under the Mental Health Act for more than two years.[26] On a day-to-day basis, when a person is behaving in a way that is seen to be 'abnormal' in public, it's unlikely that people will stop to ask whether they're diagnosed with a learning disability or a Mental Illness; but it's likely that they'll be discriminated against, excluded and policed all the same. Therefore, coming together under the 'neurodivergent' umbrella presents us with opportunities to make these links, and build coalitions against our shared oppression.

The umbrella label of 'neurodivergent' may also be useful for those of us who could be sorted into numerous diagnostic categories, or don't find it entirely useful to erect hard boundaries between one category and another. For example, many autistic people are given other psychiatric diagnoses like ADHD, OCD, PTSD, anxiety and depression. If a person is diagnosed with all of these things, are they really distinct entities? Or is a person just broadly experiencing their consciousness in a way that diverges from a socially valued norm? Waithera, a friend of mine who considers herself to be 'neurodivergent', tells me:

[Neurodivergence] is a way of acknowledging that I seem to have a different psychic experience of the world to a lot of

---

26 https://digital.nhs.uk/data-and-information/publications/statistical/learning-disability-services-statistics/at-june-2021-mhsds-april-2021-final (last accessed January 2023).

people I encounter day-to-day. It doesn't rely on labels that are ultimately shaped by the expectations of capital, and just generally fail to capture the most meaningful elements of the way I experience my bodymind . . . It's useful day-to-day because it helps me engage with my mental health by asking how the world is shaped wrongly for my brain, rather than the other way around.

The neurodiversity paradigm also presents us with alternative ways of thinking about our mental experiences, which can be useful for some. Not everyone sees mental distress or Madness as an illness, not everyone wants treatment or a cure, and, for some, treatment may simply not be an option. The neurodiversity paradigm allows us to interrogate the construct of the 'normal' mind, and binaries of healthy/ill. It also makes space for the idea that what is considered Mental Illness, in one context, might be considered a gift in another – for example, cultural and historical contexts in which people who hear voices have been seen as Shamanic, psychic or otherwise spiritually connected. The 'plural' community, that is, those that believe that they have more than one 'consciousness' or 'person' sharing a body (sometimes psychiatrically diagnosed as dissociative identity disorder), has also often found respite in the neurodiversity paradigm. Obscura, who is plural, tells me that she sees the neurodiversity paradigm as perfectly compatible with her experiences, because 'there is nothing to be ashamed of, or even really wrong or necessarily disruptive about being trans and plural.'

Another important part of the neurodiversity paradigm is its shift away from *value*. People often mistake the paradigm for suggesting that neurodivergence is always a 'superpower', or that it is incompatible with the desire to seek medication or therapy for our difficulties. This would present clear problems for people with mental health struggles, since many of us do want to reduce our distress. But the neurodiversity paradigm, at its core, rejects the idea that neurocognitive differences make us less valuable or inferior to anyone considered 'normal', and resists the notion that our existence must be 'fixed' or eradicated. There is space for us all to exist and thrive, and that means something different for everyone.

From disability rights to 'Crip' justice

Over the last few decades, political understandings of disability have shifted and evolved in both academic and activist spaces. Some people have moved towards the word 'Crip' – which is derived from an ableist slur – and therefore allows them to proudly reclaim language that has been historically used to oppress physically disabled people. By taking back a slur that is uncomfortable for many (in a similar way to the word 'queer'), 'Crip' doesn't ask for respectability or assimilation. It aims to confront and disrupt, putting disability front and centre.

'Crip' has also been taken up as a politicised identity term in the disability justice movement of the twenty-first century. This movement has a different emphasis to earlier disability activism and scholarship, which was very focused around the social model, civil rights and inclusion. 'Disability justice', however, which was formulated in 2005 by a collective including Patty Berne, Mia Mingus and Stacey Milbern, emphasises intersectionality and solidarity across disabilities and movements. The disability justice movement centres the oppression of disabled people of colour, immigrants, queer people, trans and gender non-conforming people, houseless people, incarcerated people and indigenous people.[27] Disability justice organisers and 'Crip-of-colour' scholars have, for example, taken aim at high rates of Black psychiatric incarceration; the maddening and disabling nature of borders; the fact that the eugenic notion of 'degeneracy' was used not only for Mad and disabled people, but also for Black people; and the fact that the occupation of Palestine produces disability (or 'debility').[28] They see the links between capitalism, colonialism, gendered violence and disability, and show that they cannot be disentangled.

Crip academics have also continued to challenge the idea of what disability actually *is*. In his book *Crip Theory*, the theorist Robert McRuer coined the concept of 'compulsory able-bodiedness/mindedness' – suggesting that able-bodiedness/mindedness is a constructed norm that we are all pressured to try and achieve. Even if you don't consider yourself to be disabled, McRuer argues, you are affected by the compulsion to be 'normal'. By starting with able-bodiedness/mindedness, this concept that is so normalised that it is rarely ever named, McRuer turns away from interrogating disability as an identity category, to instead interrogate the harmful system that disability exists in opposition to. Who is really 'able-bodied'? When I ask this question, I think about my older relatives, who would never call themselves 'disabled', but increasingly have a 'dodgy hip' or a 'bad leg' in the cold weather. I think of my friends who can't make their way through the world when their glasses break, the ones who always seem to be sick or run down, the ones whose backs hurt if they stand for too long, the ones who haven't had an epileptic seizure since childhood, the ones who 'haven't felt 100%' since they contracted Covid, the ones who have an injury,

27 https://resourceguides.hampshire.edu/c.php (last accessed January 2023).
28 J. K. Puar, *The Right to Maim: Debility, Capacity, Disability* (Durham, NC: Duke University Press, 2017).

the ones who aren't necessarily mentally 'well', the ones who never got a diagnosis.

While many of these people would not be recognised by the state as 'officially' disabled, they subtly diverge from the idolised concept of the 'perfect' or able bodymind in all kinds of ways. When we start to interrogate the question of who is and isn't able-bodied, we also see how many people would benefit from the things that make the world more accessible to disabled people – like public seating and toilets, the destigmatisation of mobility aids, the mass availability of these aids, unlimited sick leave, the ability to work from home, and an end to medical gatekeeping. By turning its attention to 'normality', Crip theory shows how disability, and disability justice, is relevant to everyone. It shows that, even if you have an 'able' bodymind, this identity exists only in *opposition* to disability; disability sits beyond, beneath and beside you.[29] It concerns you, and one day, it will be you. As Susan Sontag writes, everyone who is born holds dual citizenship, in the kingdom of the well and in the kingdom of the sick[30] – a reality that came to the fore during the Covid-19 pandemic, when we all had to grapple with the fragility of our bodies. If we want to hold solidarity with disabled people, our proximity to disability is something we should turn towards, rather than turn away from.

If the 'able' bodymind is a construction that almost all of us are constantly grasping towards, Crip theory also considers what it might mean to reach in the other direction. It allows us to question the idea of 'norm' as 'good', and consider other ways of embodiment. What would it mean to embrace being disabled, Mad, abnormal or deviant? Is that allowed? This

---

29   E. K. Sedgwick, *Touching Feeling: Affect, Pedagogy, Performativity* (Durham and London: Duke University Press, 2003).

30   S. Sontag, *Illness as Metaphor* (New York: Vintage Books, 1979).

impulse is something that can undoubtedly be connected to Mad movements, which, as we will discuss in later chapters, have similarly reclaimed previously stigmatised language, and tried to embrace the possibilities contained in that idea of 'disorder'. Crip theory's resistance to binary thinking and identity politics may also be useful to Mad/Mentally Ill people who feel they sit on the fringes of disability, and are unsure whether they can be a part of the movement. Disability is not always clear cut or straightforward – it can be invisible, elusive, nuanced, leaky, transient or in flux. It is worth thinking critically about these ambiguities, and acknowledging that the resultant 'imposter syndrome' is a part of the disabled experience for a significant number of people. Many of us are worried that we don't 'count', but that is no reason to shut ourselves off from the movement entirely.

Interdependence, interrelatedness

Everything on earth – from trees to rivers to bacteria – is *interdependent*, whether we realise it or not. This applies to our societies; we rely on each other to grow our food, make our clothes, deliver our letters, drive our public transport, teach our children, write our books, move our waste. However, many of these forms of interdependence are normalised and made invisible under neoliberal capitalism – we are encouraged to think of ourselves as individual, self-sufficient units. The way we arrange our lives and resources – often isolated from one another in households or nuclear family units – is conducive to this thinking. This is why, when disabled people need forms of care and support that aren't normalised within these systems, they are so often framed as 'scroungers', 'dependent', 'needy' or having 'special needs'. But we all need lots of things.

Recently, I revisited the magazine profile in which former prime minister Margaret Thatcher famously declared that there is 'no such thing as a society' – that the world is only made up of 'individual men and women'.[31] As I read on, I was struck by the less notorious quote that follows, which states that people 'must look after themselves first'; because it's exactly the sort of 'inspiring' mantra I could imagine scrolling past on social media. The concept of 'self-care' is not harmful in and of itself – it was popularised by the Black Panthers' 'survival programs' in the US, which aimed to inject health, skills and knowledge into impoverished communities. But 'self-care' has since been largely co-opted to suggest that we are not responsible for looking after one another at all.

The disability justice movement, like the Black Panthers, has embraced cultures of community care and mutual aid as a response to abandonment by the state, in order to keep one another alive. Mutual aid is not driven by pity or charity – it is about offering material support to your peers because you are all fighting against the same systems. During Covid lockdowns, this meant getting food, medications and homemade hand sanitiser to other disabled people.[32] In other contexts, it might mean making an acquaintance a care package containing things they need when they are sick; or doing admin, laundry or errands for someone when they're depressed or in crisis. My friend Lauren, who I have developed a relationship of mutual care and aid with, tells me:

Care and interdependency in Crip communities is a bit like spinning plates. We take turns to top each other up, stabilise things a little, maybe [soon] we'll start spinning dangerously,

---

31   www.margaretthatcher.org/document/106689 (last accessed January 2023).
32   https://disabilityvisibilityproject.com/2021/10/03/how-disabled-mutual-aid-is-different-than-abled-mutual-aid/ (last accessed January 2023).

but we'll get some attention back from someone who's in a good enough place to give it. We try really hard to make sure no one topples and smashes. The reality of sick interdependence, for me, is that we are all lovingly dragging each other through things, in a world that often has us on our knees.

Although myself and Lauren have different experiences of disability, we have been able to make an instinctive connection between our struggles, and offer support to each other as a result. I have seen disability bring so many others together in similar ways – allowing us to make links between experiences that appear very different on the surface. I regularly attend a Crip theory reading group, started by the academic Akanksha Mehta as a 'teach-out' during a wave of strikes at Goldsmiths University in London. In one session, we discussed the societal expectation that people should all use spoken English – and, as people brought their lived experiences forward, we found that this was an issue that impacted d/Deaf people, autistic people, dyslexic people, people who struggle to speak because of their chronic pain, non-native English speakers and many others. In moments like this, I have noticed that when people with so many different embodied experiences come together in a space, it is possible to identify unexpected sources of common exclusion. When we see that our oppression is so closely interrelated, it becomes easier to dismantle it, and build new worlds together. This capacity to make novel connections is something that people with experience of Madness/Mental Illness can undoubtedly gain from disability spaces.

Relating to disability

The choice to identify as disabled is an incredibly personal one that we can only make for ourselves. However, on a practical level, it can be a powerful means to foster solidarity across communities divided by different life experiences and diagnostic labels. In this sense, 'disabled' is not an individual fact, but what the historian Joan W. Scott describes as a 'collective affinity';[33] it provides us with a lens to describe and act upon our common oppression, in a society that wants to divide and disappear us. In a world in which one billion people might be considered disabled,[34] but far fewer identify that way, embracing the language of disability can be a form of resistance in itself. Rather than leaning into the idea that disability means we are defective or irredeemable, what if we embraced disability and Cripness as a radical disruption to political and economic systems that harm us all?

On the question of whether Mad/Mentally Ill people should call ourselves 'disabled', the answer is: the possibility is ours if we want it. But, far more urgent than the question of self-identification is how we utilise disability as a means of understanding the world, and coming together to change it. Disability is not a closing down of possibilities – on the contrary, it is a portal – an opening up of so many different ways of being, understanding and relating to the world around us. Far from being synonymous with 'broken' or 'lacking': disability is possibility.

---

33 Kafer, *Feminist, Queer, Crip*.
34 https://un.org/development/desa/disabilities/resources/factsheet-on-persons-with-disabilities.html (last accessed January 2023).

Chapter 6

Diagnosing diagnosis

Diagnosis wields immense power. It can provide us access to vital medical technology or shame us, reveal a path towards less pain or get us locked up. It opens doors and slams them shut. – Eli Clare

Resisting biocertification does not mean resisting 'diagnosis' or identification. It means resisting the leveraging of these certifications by capital and the state. – Beatrice Adler-Bolton and Artie Vierkant

This chapter contains a mention of suicide.

Emily first got a psychiatric diagnosis aged 14, and since, has been given a whole host of other labels. 'First I got diagnosed with depression, then anxiety, then social anxiety, then bipolar, and finally borderline personality disorder.' Over the course of the 15 years since her first contact with mental health services, Emily's diagnoses have changed many times, but right now, she has a dual diagnosis of bipolar type 2 and borderline personality disorder (BPD).

Emily's diagnoses are not the only thing that has changed – her relationship to the process has also evolved over time. 'I've basically done a full 180,' she tells me. 'When I first got diagnosed with depression (and later bipolar) I was really pleased.

I felt like it was a way of validating what I was experiencing, which I didn't have words for at the time.' But today, Emily, who defines as a psychiatric survivor, identifies with neither term, saying she is 'most passionately opposed to the BPD label by far.' Her rejection of diagnostic labels is challenging to the authoritative logics of both psychiatry and broader medicine – it calls into question their ability to produce 'truth'.

Diagnosis is the foundation upon which Western medicine is built. When we think about mental health, diagnosis may be one of the first things we think of – stencils that draw the perimeters of our experiences, and influence the way that so many of us think about them. But diagnosis does not reveal internal realities about our bodyminds – the true, material nature of our flesh and bones – although we often think of it this way. Diagnosis is not 'illness' itself. Rather, diagnosis is a particular lens for thinking about different bodymind states, currently dominated by a medical industrial complex that expanded in line with colonialism and eugenics, and continues to be inseparable from capitalist desires. Like each of these systems, diagnosis makes value judgments about which kinds of bodyminds are faulty, unproductive and unruly. It carries hallmarks of the past – of how medicine and psychiatry have historically sorted the 'good' people from the 'bad' ones, then further spliced the 'good' parts of bodyminds from the 'bad', dissecting us further and further. It attempts to make order and certainty out of the beauty and chaos of our bodies, societies and world. We often discuss diagnosis as an adjective (something we are) or a noun (something we have), when in actuality, diagnosis is a verb – a process by which doctors look at a set of attributes (or 'symptoms'), and choose a lens through which to gaze at us.

Diagnosis is also a prophecy. It comes bearing knowledge of how our bodyminds might change over time (how do others like me fare? Is it 'terminal', 'chronic' or 'curable'?). But it also gives us a glimpse into the future of many other social and material realities. A medical diagnosis may influence which medications and treatments become available to us, whether we are institutionalised, and how we are treated by professionals. The potential outcomes under our current conditions range from life-saving to deadly. A diagnosis of 'personality disorder', described in public correspondence by the Royal College of Psychiatrists as a 'thorn in the flesh of many clinicians,'[1] can spell particularly violent experiences with mental health services for the remainder of a person's life. Emily says that after she received a diagnosis of BPD, which often sees its bearers stereotyped as manipulative and attention-seeking, her treatment in mental health services 'significantly degraded'. 'The BPD label has affected my ability to access all kinds of care, and the way people talk to me and treat me.' In other contexts, diagnosis is the only key that unlocks the door to medication or therapy. Cameron* who has self-diagnosed with autism, ADHD and depression, tells me: '[I see it] as a means to an end to get medicated – as I'm trying to do with ADHD.'

Since illness is constructed in the shadow of production, employers, the education system and the welfare state centre diagnosis just as much as medical and psychiatric institutions. Diagnosis is the arbitrary standard we must meet – a means of 'bio-certification' – that the state uses to separate the deserving from the undeserving. You may therefore need a diagnosis to get your benefits granted or to gain other forms of government support; or to get reasonable adjustments in education. Since ideas of 'productivity' and 'fitness' stretch their tendrils

---

1   https://twitter.com/MsCatEdwards/status/1508482146205380617 (last accessed January 2023).

* Name has been changed.

into almost every domain of life, from parenthood to the border regime, diagnosis might also be the mark on your record that gets your children taken away or your citizenship denied. Diagnoses, and each of the state systems that jointly produce it, have so many potential life-saving or life-destroying outcomes. When it comes to psychiatric diagnosis – which has no blood test, no brain scan, no 'biological' measure to bolster the highly precarious and political lines drawn between each category – we are completely at the mercy of medical professionals, their opinions, their prejudices, and their whims. Psychiatric diagnoses also have low 'inter-rater reliability', meaning that the same person may get very different opinions or diagnoses from different professionals. Contrary to the popular myth that they are based on 'chemical imbalances', psychiatric diagnoses are socially decided.[2]

Diagnosis comes with specific social and cultural meanings. A diagnosis of schizophrenia produces a 'schizophrenic person' – a concept that may seem more 'knowable', but that society (and the person themselves) will carry particular expectations and judgements about. These ideas might alleviate stigma, in other cases they are a clear source of stigma. Therefore, as diagnosis solidifies knowledge, it also takes other possibilities away. These meanings may differ between labels and across time and space. A diagnosis of cancer or depression might, in some contexts, evoke pity or tenderness, while a diagnosis of schizophrenia or HIV might, in the very same context, evoke fear, exclusion and violence. We may strategically conceal and deploy diagnosis according to changing goalposts. A person with a diagnosis of autism might want to celebrate and claim it within neurodiversity communities, disclose it to the HR department to get their

2   J. Moncrieff, R. E. Cooper, T. Stockmann, et al., 'The serotonin theory of depression: a systematic umbrella review of the evidence', *Mol Psychiatry* (2022).

access needs met, and conceal it from their boss who would never treat them the same way. Therefore, debates that treat diagnosis as a noun (is diagnosis 'good' or 'bad'?) largely overlook the fact that diagnosis is a powerful and kinetic process – always moving, always serving an end. Within the current system, it can therefore be deployed to sustain life, or to produce death. Diagnoses are passports; they are not made equally, and they are elements of a state system of gatekeeping that should not exist.

Biomedicine and pathology

In a society that is structured around productivity, and, as a result, 'health', diagnosis provides us with a social token to reconcile and accept the disruptive reality of unproductive body-minds. When bodyminds become what we call 'ill', they throw a spanner into the business-as-usual factory line. In the 1950s, the conservative sociologist Talcott Parsons devised a concept called the 'sick role'. He thought that people who were (temporarily) ill were not responsible for their unproductiveness, that being ill wasn't a choice, and that sick people should be exempt from daily duties as long as they submitted to medical institutions and worked to become healthy again.[3] While we might reject Parsons' politics, he accurately describes the societal approach to people designated as ill. This is a unique social quality of 'illness', that it can make a person, *within highly conditional and specific bounds*, exempt from some 'blame' for transgressing social and economic expectations. An appeal to the amoral driving force of biology – justifying bodyminds as 'sick' rather than 'criminal', 'disordered' rather than 'lazy', 'born this way' rather than inten-tionally deviant – may offer some respite. This takes place in

---

3   T. Parsons, *The Social System* (London: Routledge, 1951).

the context of a punishing world that holds individuals morally responsible for socially constructed transgressions like 'crime' or 'laziness'. Illness offers an alternative explanation to moral blame. This was the case for Emily when she first received her bipolar diagnosis – she tells me: 'Because I had been blamed and stigmatised for periods of mania or depression, the idea that I was "ill" rather than a "bad person" was really powerful for me, having internalised so many of those sanist narratives.'

There is, however, always a catch. This biological and medical (biomedical) framing of our suffering and disability, which suggests that it emanates from some bodily dysfunction disconnected from the social world, is a medical construct, which can also produce blame. In recent decades, there has been a push in both psychiatry and broader medicine towards a 'biopsychosocial' model, which claims to take account of the biological, psychological and social factors of illness. In practice, however, the focus of Western modern medicine remains individualistic[4] – and focused on the failure of our bodyminds to meet social and economic demands. Interactions with GPs take place in sterile, isolated rooms, behind closed doors, entirely removed from our day-to-day social contexts. Research and funding is poured into profitable pharmaceutical and technological interventions, bolstering the promise that doctors will be able to see further and further into our bodyminds, revealing and tweaking newfound 'chemical imbalances' and 'dysfunctions' as they go. Diagnosis is therefore still largely biomedical in the way that it is performed and understood, and also in the solutions that it offers for our suffering.

I was recently diagnosed with vitamin D deficiency, which usually results from lack of exposure to sunlight, and was told

---

4   J. Read, 'The bio-bio-bio model of madness', *The Psychologist*, 18, (2005), p. 596.

I should be taking the supplement for the rest of my life. The reasons I didn't get enough access to the sun – my work-from-home desk job, my overwhelm, my lack of access to a garden – were social and economic problems outside of the doctor's remit. Therefore the doctor's biomedical lens obscured these issues, and attempted to remedy the 'problem' inside my body. Biomedical psychiatry similarly squeezes social problems through a narrow, individualistic lens, obscuring the clearly social, political and economic drivers of mass suffering. For example, the diagnosis of clinical depression spans a near-infinite number of experiences. If you ask a person with this diagnosis about the context of their feelings, you will undoubtedly hear an entirely unique story that differs from the next person.[5] Some people might talk about poverty or poor working conditions, others, about their immigration status, others, still, an abusive relationship, others, loneliness. Therefore, the transformation of complex social experience into diagnostic language may mute our political realities. In the same vein, it can serve as a smokescreen for various forms of violence. When people die by suicide while waiting for benefits or for trans healthcare, suicide may be read as a result of illness that originated from inside the person's mind. The state's responsibility for social murder is therefore diminished. This process of medicalisation also leads the living towards overwhelmingly medical 'solutions' for distress; we are prescribed drugs or cognitive behavioural therapy (CBT) instead of revolution.

For Emily, these political limits of the biomedical framework are what initially led her to move away from diagnosis as a means of understanding herself:

---

5   L. Fannen, *Warp And Weft: Psycho-Emotional Health, Politics And Experiences* (n.p.: Active Distribution, 2021).

In my mid-twenties, I started to read about and get involved in the survivor movement, and came across different models of health that started to make more sense to me. The social model of disability was huge for me here – I honestly found it revelatory in the way that it shifted my understanding of things.

Emily also went into psychoanalysis, with an analyst who was extremely non-medical in their outlook, and started to look at the role of social phenomena in her life, like trauma. This kind of in-depth exploration is particularly pertinent for many people diagnosed with BPD, since it is overwhelmingly diagnosed in women and trauma survivors.[6,7] Emily says: 'Looking at these factors started to make much more sense to me than the idea that there was something wrong with my brain chemistry.'

The biomedical and pathological framing also suppresses the fact that there is no 'correct', 'natural' or 'right' type of bodymind – it doesn't exist. Of course, there are bodymind states that bring about more or less suffering, that we might want to change, that stop us from doing things we want to, that lead us to die earlier than we might do otherwise. But the idea that these are natural categories, and that there is some ultimate 'healthy' bodymind that we should always be striving towards, is a Western, medical, capitalist fiction. People choose states labelled as 'illness' all the time, and doing so may feel subversive or liberating, particularly within a medical framework that has pathologised oppressed people's responses to, and dissent against, the conditions of their society.

6   A.E. Skodol, D.S. Bender, 'Why are women diagnosed borderline more than men?', *Psychiatric Quarterly*, 74(4), (2003), pp. 349–60.

7   C. Porter, J. Palmier-Claus, A. Branitsky, W. Mansell, H. Warwick, and F. Varese, 'Childhood Adversity and Borderline Personality Disorder: A Meta-Analysis', Acta *Psychiatrica Scandinavica*, 141(1), (2020), pp. 6–20.

A non-pathologising framing was central to the anti-psychiatry and psychiatric survivor movements of the late twentieth century. In the 1970s, the US-based psychiatric survivor journal Madness Network News rejected the term 'Mental Illness', stating that they 'did not believe that psychiatric survivors had any particular illness or mental impairment'.[8] Into the 1990s, the 'Mad Pride' movement, which centred around the reclamation and celebration of Madness, further popularised the approach. These groups emphasised Madness as a human difference or a positive form of identity. In the new millennium, a US peer support network called the Icarus Project described Madness as a 'dangerous gift'[9] – which needed to be cultivated and taken care of, rather than treated as a disease to be cured. Many people diagnosed with bipolar have argued that they would not change it if given the choice[10] – for example, Kay Redfield Jamison has written:

> As a result of [bipolar] I have felt more things, more deeply; had more experiences, more intensely . . . I have seen the breadth and depth and width of my mind and heart and seen how frail they both are, and how ultimately *unknowable* they both are [emphasis added].[11,12]

Indigenous approaches to healing also show us what life could look like outside of Western pathology. The Mad Crip care worker Stefanie Lyn Kaufman-Mthimkhulu writes of how her

8 https://madinamerica.com/2021/01/madness-network-news/ (last accessed January 2023).

9 J. Bossewitch, *Dangerous Gifts*, (Thesis, Columbia University, 2016).

10 See Stephen Fry's documentary, *The Secret Life of the Manic Depressive*.

11 K. Redfield Jamison, *An Unquiet Mind: A Memoir of Moods and Madness* (London: Pan Macmillan, 2014).

12 Crucially, however, Jamison says that she would only do so if she could keep using lithium as medication.

partner Thabiso Mthimkhulu, an Afro-indigenous ancestral healer, would respond to a person who was hearing voices. His approach centred around putting the voice in context, and looking for its symbolic meaning. For example, if a person was hearing the voice of a baby crying, he might approach the person's loved ones to find out if they lost a baby, or what was happening when they were a baby.[13] He says that he would also connect with the person's ancestors, to ask: 'Does this person need to be born again, spiritually? Are they hearing the sounds of themselves crying as a child? What does this child need to communicate?'[14] This approach, similarly to the philosophies of the Mad movement, reveals the limits of biomedical framings, which do not make space for the many potential social interpretations of Madness.

Who has the power?

It is easy to forget that diagnosis, in its current form, is a system of state power. We do not get final say in the terminology that is applied to our bodyminds. In a society in which we ascribe such weight to the authority of the medical industrial complex, this idea is incredibly normalised, despite the fact that most diagnosis could not take place without Mad/disabled knowledge. For those of us who have had positive and consensual diagnosis experiences, we should ask ourselves: how much of the process was really performed by professionals alone? Most of us have some idea of what our 'symptoms' are before we set foot in the doctor's office; we often know what treatment we want too. When we first have a symptom or complaint, it is commonplace

---

13   https://medium.com/@stefkaufman/visions-for-a-liberated-anti-carceral-crisis-response-c81791459a99 (last accessed January 2023).
14   Ibid.

to go to Google, read online forums and crowdsource information before ever engaging with medical institutions. If we do
engage with them, disabled people often go to get second, third
and fourth opinions afterwards – which is a type of investiga-
tory work in itself. Trans, sick and disabled people often share
their experiences in accessing diagnosis, so others can rehearse
exactly what they must say to doctors to get the care that they
need. People are also often denied useful diagnoses because they
are Black, Fat,[15] poor, Mad/Mentally Ill, or don't meet other arbitrary metrics of deservingness. Doctors do not have a monopoly
on the process of diagnosis – or, rather, of *identification*. They
may hoard training, technologies, literature and other resources
within the institution, and give the final rubber stamp for the
purposes of the state. But positive identification processes
are often actually collectively made in the community. This is
particularly significant in the realm of mental health, where
diagnosis is not grounded in biomarkers, is often wielded violently, and, on its own, actually has little bearing on treatment
options.

For Emily, power has played a significant role in the many
diagnoses she has been given over the course of 15 years. 'I've
basically had no say in what labels I've been given or how I'm
treated because of them. Fundamentally, psychiatrists have the
power to diagnose you no matter what you think or say, and that
power relation then iterates itself over and over again within
other relationships with professionals.' These power dynamics
are particularly exaggerated in psychiatry, because diagnoses
are frequently dispensed under non-consensual conditions, for
example, when people are detained under the Mental Health
Act. Neha, who at age 15 was diagnosed with schizoaffective

---

15 I use this term in line with Fat thinkers, who have reclaimed the word as a
neutral descriptor.

disorder without her knowledge or consent while detained on a psychiatric ward, tells me that she only found out about it three years later, when she requested her notes. 'I was pretty shocked and upset when I found out . . . I felt like I'd been lied to for no real reason other than that they couldn't be bothered to explain it to me . . . [I felt] very scared and alone.'

On the ward, diagnoses may be used to further justify violations of consent – under the logic that people 'must' be restrained, forcibly drugged, secluded or otherwise punished because they are 'sick'. The scholar Eunjung Kim calls this 'curative violence', 'when cure is what actually frames the presence of disability as a problem and ends up destroying the subject in the curative process . . . [becoming] at once remedy and poison'.[16] Professionals can also use their power to pathologise people's responses to this violence, resulting in further dehumanisation and delegitimisation. When people become distressed, self-harm, argue or try to defend themselves against their mistreatment, these responses may be medicalised by professionals as signs of deteriorating illness. Their diagnosis becomes a trump card – nothing a person says or does is immune to becoming a 'symptom'. This also plays out on the outside in the form of epistemic injustice. People may, for example, question whether they can trust the testimony of a psychiatric survivor with a diagnosis of schizophrenia, because they are seen as an unreliable narrator of their own experiences.

Self-knowledge, community knowledge and language

Many people who choose to identify with psychiatric diagnoses have argued that one of its most important elements is entirely

---

16   E. Kim, *Curative Violence: Rehabilitating Disability, Gender, and Sexuality in Modern Korea* (Durham, NC: Duke University Press, 2017).

separate to the mental health system. As a type of language, diagnoses provide many people with common tools to communicate their experiences with others. Diagnostic categories may be constructed, but this doesn't mean these experiences, and the material conditions that construct them, aren't 'real'. Therefore many do find that diagnostic terminology goes some way to describing their lived realities. It may provide us with words to articulate exactly how and why the structures of work and society exclude us, and to describe the specific contours of our suffering. For some, terms like PTSD are also a very useful shorthand when communicating with professionals, new people or employers, sparing us from having to delve into and disclose personal or traumatic information. These are uses of diagnosis that can be leveraged to work for us as individuals, rather than simply for the state.

Autonomy is also central to the spirit of 'self-diagnosis', a process by which people self-identify with diagnostic terminology without (or in spite of) professional opinion. Self-diagnosis works upon the principle that state, medical or psychiatric authority is not a precursor to understanding ourselves. It actively dissents against their monopoly on identification, and undermines the idea that the state has the final say in describing our bodyminds. It also imagines diagnosis beyond the institution, providing a glimpse into how communities might reclaim and democratise medical knowledge, processes, resources and technologies. Self-diagnosis may allow us to avoid the state violence that can result from 'official' diagnosis. It may blend institutional knowledge with the wisdom of Mad/Mentally Ill communities, disabled communities and indigenous traditions. It may also help us find others who share the same experiences, allowing us to cluster in our own decentralised communities and opening up opportunities for solidarity, care, support, exploration and discovery. Communities that practise self-diagnosis also often actively reject biomedical approaches. For example, autistic communities have asserted that 'autism' describes a broad cluster of very real experiences of the world, not a discrete or objective biological disorder. When people are denied diagnosis or healthcare, community spaces that value self-diagnosis may offer a place to share tips, to better understand our shared oppression, and to organise against it. They turn diagnosis into a tool for solidarity rather than individualism.

Those of us who wholly reject our diagnoses may still participate in similar processes of self-identification. Emily tells me:

> I do see myself as part of a community with other people diagnosed with BPD, but I relate to that less in terms of symptoms and more in terms of being a political class who are subject to many of the same powers and discourses as each other. For this reason I tend to tell people 'I have a diagnosis of BPD' rather than 'I have/am BPD', to try to highlight my material position within mental health services while also rejecting the fact of the diagnosis itself.

She says that involvement in communities of people with similar experiences – whether they identify with or reject the BPD label – has been extremely healing, as they share common experiences of injustice within mental health services.

It is deeply important that communities of self-identification do not replicate essentialist ideas, become just another form of liberal identity politics, and sweep people into diagnosis-based silos devoid of solidarity between one another. Diagnosis should not be a kind of property ownership. For this reason, Cameron says that they do not form community based on diagnosis alone:

I share experiences with people of the same and different diagnoses, and part of what makes disability community so rich is its foundational diversity of experience – I don't need to share symptoms, diagnoses, or precise types of same experience to be in disability community with others who are disabled by society. I'm also very politically committed both to cross-impairment, cross-difference and cross-disability community and politics.

As Cameron asserts, a focus on personal identity labels must not distract us from addressing the social, political and economic conditions that harm us all. And it doesn't have to; many use a combination of language that feels more personal and more political in tandem, for example, simultaneously identifying with both 'PTSD' and 'Madness'.

Moving with, against, and beyond diagnosis

Diagnosis is a tool. Its utility and its violence can't be viewed in a vacuum – they speak to the power dynamics entrenched in psychiatry, and the broader failures of biomedical frameworks to genuinely respond to human suffering and difference. As we have established throughout the course of this book so far, biomedical approaches are blinkered and inadequate lenses for collectively understanding and caring for our bodyminds. They are rooted in murky histories, they turn our attention away from the political world, and obscure the ways in which our societal context constructs illness and disability.

Nonetheless, Mad/Mentally Ill people who share these criticisms of diagnosis have come to different conclusions about what to do with it. Some reject all diagnostic language, some see it as just one piece of the puzzle, and others take it into collective ownership and transform its meaning. All are united in their rejection of a solely biomedical approach. Regardless of which approach we choose to take, I believe that the ability to define ourselves and our suffering must be collectively placed into the hands of the people most affected. This means dismantling artificial divisions between expertise versus lived experience, practitioner versus patient, good knowledge versus bad knowledge, healthy versus ill. There are so many different ways that this could look. It might mean rejecting diagnosis in favour of other explanations, if that feels right for you. It might look like claiming it, if you think it has utility as an explanation for your experience in the world, and brings you together with others. It might look like reclaiming it – taking labels that often work against us, seizing control of them and reshaping them as political categories that work for us instead. Or it might look like a combination of the above.

We can resist the power of the medical and psychiatric industrial complexes to dictate identification, all the while allowing space for people to name their experiences in the way that makes most sense for them. In dreaming towards this reality, we should look to those who are already navigating life beyond diagnosis; for example, the trans communities that have had to bypass medicine and create their own underground access to life-saving treatments.[17] Crucially, these communities prioritise self-identification and self-determination over categories enforced by the state.

Moving beyond fierce and divisive debates around diagnosis requires a kind of Mad, radical and utopian thinking. Would diagnosis matter so much in a society in which everyone could get what they needed, without requiring proof? A system of

17   https://thebaffler.com/salvos/doctors-who-gill-peterson (last accessed January 2023).

social organisation in which trans healthcare, mental health medication and all other healing processes centred informed consent, rather than medical gatekeeping?[18] One that valued life over bureaucracy? A world in which expertise and testing were not confined to institutional power structures? One in which we could describe our experiences however we wanted? What new types of language and identification might bloom in such a world? Ultimately, diagnosis is characterised by power and gatekeeping. This is the process that we must take aim at and dismantle. We should build towards a future where communities can lead research and exploration, and collectively devise ways of describing ourselves and relating to one another that are characterised by creativity, complexity, community, abundance and solidarity. We may create pathways, maps and ways of thinking about how different bodily experiences progress, and ways of responding to them too. But this transformed kind of diagnosis or self-identification should be produced collectively, free from state control. This future is uncertain and could take a number of forms, but it must be one where diagnosis can never again be the difference between care and punishment, life and death.

18   https://devonprice.medium.com/toward-an-informed-consent-model-for-all-drugs-9106aff593a4 (last accessed January 2023).

Chapter 7

On disavowal and disorder

The rejection of rhetorics of disorder . . . is never innocent of the very processes of stigmatization that speakers or thinkers are trying to renounce. – Robert McRuer

All sickness is essentially deviancy. – Peter Sedgwick

Disorder is a construct, like everything else. This doesn't mean that it isn't real, or that the overwhelming pain and anguish that often falls under its remit are fictional. Rather, it means that the concept is shaped by the social world, that it is hard to define, and that its boundaries are murky and unstable.

The boundaries that designate particular bodyminds as disordered, diseased, disabled or deviant are social and economic, and have been drawn and redrawn across historical and cultural contexts. Doctors in Victorian England considered menstruation to be a monthly illness that disabled women.[1] Old age has slowly become more and more medicalised across history; osteoporosis, for example, which used to be considered a 'normal' part of ageing, was declared as a disease by the World Health Organisation (WHO) in 1994.[2] As Fat people are continually demonised in our society, medicine increasingly seeks to control

---

1   https://tandfonline.com/doi/pdf/10.1080/09612020000200260 (last accessed January 2023).

2   J. L. Scully, 'What is a disease?' *EMBO Reports*, 5:7, (2004), pp. 650–53.

people's size too, endorsing arbitrary cut-off points for 'healthy' weight, and suggesting that obesity should be officially recognised as a disease.[3] The concepts of illness, disease and disorder are shaped by social and economic values regarding what is normal versus abnormal, desirable versus undesirable,[4] productive versus unproductive.

Due to the constructed nature of disorder, disease, disability and deviance, there is a rich history of marginalised groups rejecting medicalisation. Members of the d/Deaf community, people with dwarfism, Fat people, intersex people and colonised people have long resisted their categorisation as deviant or disordered – asserting that there is nothing objectively or inherently wrong with their bodyminds. Many members of these communities have argued that it is society that has labelled them as deviant, that they are only seen as disordered because their bodyminds do not suit the arbitrary demands of the capitalist mode of production, that social barriers like language and architecture disable them, and that they have their own thriving cultures and communities outside of the dominant order. When eugenicist thought has argued that they must be eradicated or 'fixed', they have responded that it is the world that needs to radically change.

Gay men and lesbians are part of this tradition – in the early 1970s, they picketed and stormed the stage at the American Psychiatric Association's (APA) annual conference until psychiatrists eventually voted to take homosexuality out of the DSM.[5] This move helped solidify the idea that gay people were not sick and in need of 'cure' via torturous non-consensual conversion therapies, rather, it was heterosexist and homophobic society that

---

3 https://bmj.com/content/366/bmj.l4258 (last accessed January 2023).

4 Sedgwick, *PsychoPolitics*.

5 https://daily.jstor.org/how-lgbtq-activists-got-homosexuality-out-of-the-dsm/ (last accessed January 2023).

was the sickness. Today, many LGBTQ+ people still often argue for acceptability and assimilation by emphasising that they are not Mad or diseased. These arguments frequently lapse into the refrain that LGBTQ+ identities are a *normal*, *natural* and therefore *healthy* part of the world (some have even deployed evidence of 'gay animals' in the animal kingdom to secure their humanity).

The danger in these appeals to nature and normality is that they further reify deviance and disorder as something that is objective, and inherently negative. The declaration that 'we're not sick/crazy' is often followed by a derogatory 'like *them*'.[6] In arguing that we are natural and normal, we often uncritically suggest that 'naturalness' and 'normality' are things to strive towards, while simultaneously distancing ourselves from those *other* unnatural and abnormal people 'over there'.[7] We also have to endorse the idea that their unnaturalness and abnormality is something entirely objective, and that we were simply sorted into this undesirable category by mistake. When we do each of the above things, we break potential ties of solidarity with other oppressed people, in order to gain something for ourselves – in other words, we disavow them.

The disability activist Lydia X. Z. Brown has said: 'We all learn disavowal from a young age. [. . .] In order to claim our own humanity, we must always do so at the expense of somebody else . . . we do it even in the most progressive and radical of movements.'[8] It's what people do when they suggest that they are not

---

6   R. McRuer, 'No future for Crips: Disorderly conduct in the New World Order; or, Disability Studies on the verge of a nervous breakdown', *Culture—Theory—Disability: Encounters between Disability Studies and Cultural Studies*, (eds) A. Waldschmidt, H. Berressem and M. Ingwersen (Bielefeld: Transcript Verlag, 2017), pp. 63–77.

7   R. Thorneycroft, 'Crip Theory and Mad Studies: Intersections and points of departure', *Canadian Journal of Disability Studies*, 9, (2020), pp. 91–121.

8   https://vimeo.com/showcase/7186498/video/265431779 (last accessed January 2023).

like other women, other Black people, other disabled people, and so on – or when they seek to distance themselves from other marginalised groups who they might otherwise share a struggle with. Brown says:

> I [have] heard folks with physical disabilities say out loud, while I'm standing there, 'I may have a wheelchair, I may be paralyzed, I may be blind but my mind works fine'. . . And I'm standing there like, you do realize that I'm right here? I am actually certifiably crazy and actually developmentally disabled. I'm right here.[9]

The motivation to disavow is not a mystery – it is a survival instinct that may emerge when we lack the tools to address the broader structures that harm all of us. It may also result from the oppressive ideas that we all internalise about marginalised groups. However, when we disavow others in the quest for respectability, we (often inadvertently) reinforce their oppression.

The risks of such a strategy may sound abstract, but they have been concretely borne out in the history of our movements. For example, the anti-psychiatry movement of the 1960s saw collaboration between queer activists and psychiatric survivors. In fact, the delineations between the two groups were blurry, since many queer people *were* survivors of pathologisation and attempted 'treatment' by psychiatry. The two groups drew common links between their oppression. They also used these observations to argue that psychiatry was not an objective endeavour, but an institution that was infused with oppressive societal values about how our minds should be. However, when homosexuality was depathologised in 1973, the ties between these two movements

---

9   Ibid.

were largely broken. What's more, when psychiatry conceded that the inclusion of homosexuality in the DSM was some sort of error, it was able to regain some of its legitimacy as an 'objective' science, despite the fact that transphobic entries like 'transvestitism' were still included in the DSM.[10] What is often historically framed as a 'victory' for gay activists was, simultaneously, a disavowal of trans people and Mad/Mentally Ill people.[11] Today, gay people are far less likely to be forced into conversion therapy, but the movement largely didn't continue to protest against compulsory treatment for Mad/Mentally Ill people.

The potential for disavowal, however, doesn't end there. The anti-psychiatry movement also frequently disavowed sick and disabled people in its rhetoric.[12] For example, some parts of the anti-psychiatry and psychiatric survivor movements have argued that Madness or mental distress is not really an illness, because medical illnesses are natural, objective and apolitical categories.[13] When people argue that Madness/distress isn't a disorder because distressed people are not inherently broken, they also suggest that people with physical diagnoses *are* inherently broken – a logic that the disabled people's movement has been resisting for over half a century. When anti-psychiatrists have argued that people in distress should not be institutionalised because they are 'not sick or disabled', they have implied that it is

10   A. J. Lewis, '"We are certain of our own insanity": Antipsychiatry and the Gay Liberation Movement, 1968–1980', *Journal of the History of Sexuality*, 25:1, (2016), pp. 83–113.

11   For a discussion of how this links to trans liberation struggles, see Harry Josephine Giles' writing: https://nsun.org.uk/transitioning-out-of-psychiatry (last accessed January 2023).

12   A.J. Withers, 'Disability, Divisions, Definitions, and Disablism: When Resisting Psychiatry Is Oppressive', *Psychiatry Disrupted: Theorising Resistance and Crafting the (R)evolution*, B. Burstow, B.A. LeFrançois and S. Diamond (eds.), (Montreal and Kingston: McGill-Queen's University Press, 2014), 114–28.

13   Some have also rejected the label of 'disability' on these grounds.

legitimate to institutionalise sick and disabled people. And when members of these struggles say that Madness/distress cannot be an illness because it is simply a response to our oppressive society, this overlooks the fact that capitalism and oppression produces much of the world's physical sickness and disability. All disability, illness and suffering is deeply political, and each of these groups deserve liberation. Disabled movements have also at times been guilty of the same kind of disavowal – distancing themselves from the unpalatability of Madness/Mental Illness in an effort to gain respectability and rights. This mutual disavowal helps no one.

When we resist medical control, we must ensure that we do not advocate for the medical control of others. It is possible to argue against the dominant medical approach to Madness/ Mental Illness without adding credibility to the dominant medical approach to broader disorder, disease or disability. Simultaneously, it is also possible to fight for disabled rights without disavowing anyone perceived as Mad/Mentally Ill. This is about injecting subtlety and solidarity into our understanding of 'disorder' – but the impact of this nuance is significant. By connecting our struggles and standing shoulder to shoulder, we refuse to disavow one another. These forms of solidarity with 'disorderly' people can ripple further out to other members of the 'surplus class' – which includes all those deemed to be disruptive to the capitalist system. For example, we should stand by people who are criminalised, rather than arguing that Mad/ Mentally Ill people should be treated better, because they 'aren't criminals'.[14] We must continue to ask: what do each of us share with one another under the capitalist economic system? How can we liberate one another?

---

14   https://madnessnetworknews.com/2022/07/26/anti-psychiatry-vs-psychiatric-abolition/ (last accessed January 2023).

In the sphere of mental health, different activist movements have taken different approaches to disorderliness. As discussed in the previous chapter, many psychiatric survivors have rejected illness and embraced the label of Mad – reclaiming a term that has historically marked them out as deviant. Others, for example, the Socialist Patients' Collective (SPK), chose to claim the label of illness, as an umbrella term that united people across a range of experiences of pain, suffering and medical control. Adopting a Marxist viewpoint, they argued that we are *all* ill under capitalism, and that trying to divide ourselves up (by diagnoses, or by binaries like mental/physical or sick/healthy) only served to fracture us. Both approaches are united in acknowledging that disorder is a social construct – and in trying, in some way, to simultaneously reject and embrace it.[15] They acknowledge disorder as a mark of oppression and suffering, but also, conflictingly, as something that can be claimed and used for political struggles. It's there in the name: dis-*orderly* as a disruption to the status quo, dis-*ease* as agitation against the capitalist exploitation of our bodies, *deviance* as going down a different path, by choice or by coincidence. SPK, specifically, argued that we could harness this quality and 'turn illness into a weapon'.[16] Whatever approach a person might choose, we should bear in mind both the harm *and* the utility of disorder; the need to resist our oppression, while simultaneously resisting the urge to disavow others. There is so much potential to join forces between Mad/Mentally Ill, disabled, queer, trans, Fat, colonised and otherwise 'disorderly' bodyminds. We must ensure that we don't push others into the darkness as we try to struggle into the light.

---

15 Thorneycroft, 'Crip Theory and Mad Studies: Intersections and points of departure'.

16 Sozialistisches Patientenkollektiv, *SPK – Turn Illness into a Weapon for Agitation.*

Chapter 8

Art as a Mad liberation tool

This chapter contains a mention of suicide and discussions of self-harm.

Art offers us a brief respite from the drudgery of daily life. In a world that demands productivity, sanity and rationality, art is a space where our imaginations and our Madness can run riot. Artists have always had a historical association with Madness and suffering – from writers like Sylvia Plath, who died by suicide, to painters like Vincent Van Gogh, who heard voices, self-injured and believed things that others did not. Societally, we don't know what to do with their Madness; sometimes, it is framed as the origin of their creativity, other times, it is an unfortunate by-product. It is neither possible, nor desirable to diagnose the relationship between art and Madness/Mental Illness, only to note that it has been recognised for as long as they have both existed. Art clearly has a lot to offer to Madness, and Madness has a lot to offer to art.

Art can undoubtedly be a therapeutic release. Over the last century, talking therapies have prevailed as the most 'legitimate' way to express our suffering – but this one-size-fits-all approach inevitably excludes people, for example, those of us who face various communication barriers. Sophie, a friend of mine who used to run 'art for mental health' workshops, says:

Being neurodivergent, I'm quite chaotic when I create, jumping back and forth between different areas and sections. But, unlike when I'm trying to communicate to someone in real time, that's ok when making art . . . when collaging, it's a strength to bring together seemingly unrelated images to form new narratives.

Meanwhile, for those of us who have been in contact with many different professionals over the years, it is easy to become either overwhelmed or flattened by the process of repeating our stories over and over again, within the formulaic package of a legible story. Art offers freedom from these confines – a different language and perspective.

Even when we find ourselves too distressed to create something, the act of engaging with and interpreting the artistic creations of others can be deeply comforting. Sophie tells me: 'It can help us feel less alone, and be a point of connection with others. There's also something powerful about [. . .] someone capturing a feeling or experience you haven't been able to pin down, and creating something that absorbs and transforms you.' Many of us have stories of the music that has got us through the hardest days of our life, the poems, books, films or zines that make us feel less isolated in crisis. These materials are often available to us in moments where the guarded and gatekept resources within the mental health system are entirely out of reach. This makes it all the more perplexing that the healing power of art is often dismissed as somehow lacking or unscientific.

Art's emotional potential – its unashamed embrace of the *messiness of feeling* – undoubtedly represents a radical political challenge to scientific authority. It asks us to take seriously our messiest experiences, beyond the individualistic, clinical and controlled language of the lab. It defies measurement, categorisation and replication, the most revered pillars of science. The illogic and disorder of art exists in opposition to the logic and order of psychiatry. As Anna Harpin writes: 'Where the DSM is (or seeks to be) categorical, objective, static, certain, neutral, and concerned with surface behaviours, art is dimensional, relational, dynamic, uncertain, affective, and occupied with depth of experience.'[1] While art can easily be dismissed as unproductive, irrational and subjective, that is exactly where its power lies.

Blueprint, the mental health magazine that I used to edit, had a large focus on art. It felt important that readers who might be depleted, having a meltdown or in crisis, could engage with shapes and colour without authoritative direction or a linear argument. When I connect with Hel Spandler, editor of radical mental health magazine *Asylum* over a video call, they tell me that their thinking with their magazine has always been similar:

> With text, you often have to force yourself into a particular linear logic. But imagery is more three dimensional. It's also less binary as you can have a variety of vantage points sitting side by side, and you don't have to resolve those tensions. That feels important when we are often presented with overly simplified binary choices – like pro or anti diagnosis, pro or anti medication.

Imagery can also take on a fourth dimension – beyond the page – reproducing itself to be reinterpreted in different contexts, again and again. For example, Spandler tells me about a piece by Dolly Sen that graced the cover of *Asylum*: a soft red heart with overlapping edges, inscribed in lower case with the words: 'pathologise this'. With two simple words and a globally recognisable symbol, Sen's piece speaks to a thousand different ideas about loving one another, but also the ways that pathologisation

---

1   A. Harpin, *Madness, Art, and Society: Beyond Illness* (London: Routledge, 2018).

fails to respect our boundaries, even daring to encroach on our hearts and souls. The magazine editors made badges out of the artwork, and some people proudly wore them into their assessments with psychiatrists.

Fictional stories, real issues

Storytelling gives us a space to hash out different realities. Stories allow us to delve into scenarios that are simultaneously familiar and alien to us, to communicate with others, and to make political claims about the world. There are countless examples of demonising portrayals of Madness/Mental Illness in different fictional formats. Horror stories in the nineteenth and early twentieth centuries often surrounded the architectural embodiment of Madness – the lunatic asylum. These settings were presented as terrifying places for terrifying people. Into the second half of the twentieth century, films that have since been deemed as modern classics, like Alfred Hitchcock's *Psycho*, Jonathan Demme's *Silence of the Lambs* and Mary Harron's *American Psycho*, moved away from the asylum and riffed on the idea of the psychologically dangerous killer unleashed upon white middle-class Americans.

Other stories have directly undercut these narratives, showing us what Madness, and the asylum itself, really looks like from the inside. In the 1960s, Ken Kesey's novel *One Flew Over the Cuckoo's Nest* and Sylvia Plath's semi-autobiographical novel *The Bell Jar* both brought anti-psychiatry critiques to the mainstream. In each story (the former, adapted into a film by Miloš Forman), the protagonists become acquainted with the horrors of mid-century mental hospitals, and are both subjected to electroconvulsive therapy (ECT). While the mental hospital remained a terrifying setting in both narratives, the position of the mental patient was no longer a source of terror.

In *One Flew Over the Cuckoo's Nest*, protagonist Randle McMurphy (played in the film by Jack Nicholson) blurs the lines between patient and criminal, Mad and sane. The former prisoner, who finds his way into a psychiatric hospital to avoid his sentence, doesn't consider himself to be Mad/Mentally Ill, but someone who has made a lucky escape into a gentler state system. However, on the ward, McMurphy finds that, in some ways, his conditions are worse than in prison. He levels anti-psychiatry critiques towards fellow patients and staff, arguing that patients are 'no crazier than the average asshole walking around in the streets'. Meanwhile, the ward's cold, authoritarian attendant, Nurse Ratched (Louise Fletcher), represents the cartoonishly evil face of psychiatric control. The story, which is based on Kesey's own experience working as an orderly in a hospital, deeply impacted public perceptions of psychiatry,[2] as well as my own. Almost 50 years after its release, the film still immerses, enrages and moves me – reminding me of the power art has to develop our political consciousness about mental health.

Challenging power through zines

Decades after the height of the anti-psychiatry movement, many fringe art forms still possess a powerful ability to subvert hegemonic ideas. Zines – defined as 'noncommercial, nonprofessional, small-circulation magazines which their creators produce, publish and distribute by themselves'[3] – have a political history, and continued political potential. These pamphlets, which may

---

2 Shorter, *A History of Psychiatry*.

3 S. Duncombe, 'Notes from Underground: Zines and the Politics of Alternative Culture', (London: Verso, 1997).

contain illustrations, collages, photographs, comic strips and text, show how art can thrive in the margins even when deprived of finances, publishers or institutional backing. Zines are traditionally DIY in nature, with small audiences and budgets, and so have naturally flourished in liberation movements and counter-cultures. Activist zine-makers, like 'riot grrrl' feminist punks in the 1990s, have historically been able to circumvent the gatekeepers and systemic barriers found in professional arts and media industries. After all, anyone with a piece of paper and a pen can make one.

The accessibility and political independence of the form creates opportunities to challenge psychiatric power. As discussed in Chapters 2 and 6, Mad/Mentally Ill people experience 'epistemic injustice'[4] – to mean that their testimonies and beliefs are routinely dismissed as illegitimate forms of knowledge, by virtue of the fact that they are not sane. These forms of lived experience and knowledge will never hold up when weighed against that of able-minded people, professionals, and other seemingly more reliable 'knowers'. However, when I have pored through the zines of other Mad/Mentally Ill people and psychiatric survivors, I have found radical counter-narratives to mainstream mental health knowledge. Often, these new forms of knowledge will resist certainty and authority, instead opting for fluidity, ambivalence and nuance.

For example, psychiatry tends to approach self-harm as a solely negative symptom, which should be forcibly prevented at all costs, and has no internal meaning. This approach lacks curiosity and understanding, and speaks down to people. However, a number of zines about self-harm focus on harm minimisation, rather than straightforwardly advising people not to self-injure, or reprimanding people who self-harm. Self-harm zines may

---

4   Fricker, *Epistemic Injustice*.

share information on safer ways of self-harming, how to know when an injury is life-threatening, or how to care for or hide scars. Zine creators also frequently discuss the thoughts and feelings that lead to self-harm, and understand self-harm as a coping mechanism. In *(Still) Healing*, a zine about coping with and healing from self-harm, writer and illustrator Dogs Not Diets writes: 'Self-harming is dangerous and I'd love for it to never hurt anyone ever, but I know that it does so I am making this zine to support anyone to stay as safe as possible when staying safe is impossible'. This message doesn't come from a place of authority or discipline, but one of lived experience and solidarity. The writer adds: 'I get that when it's the only thing that seems to help you cope, people telling you that you must stop is both annoying and just not a possibility'.

While some people might see this framing as irresponsible or risky, it points towards a fundamental distinction between medicine and radical art forms. While medicine is clinical, pre-scriptive and aims to dictate authoritative truths toward passive subjects, art embraces complexity and multiplicity, and offers up agency, nuance and subjectivity to the person interpreting it. In their zine, Dogs Not Diets adds: 'as with all these tips, what works for me may be the opposite of what is helpful to you.' This tailored guidance resists a 'production line' approach to mental health; we are all individuals, and we all need very different things out of our care, which only we can know. While psychiatry aims to issue seamless blanket guidance, zines are what zine-maker and researcher Paula Cameron has described as 'seamful'[5] – they are messy, and show their workings.

---

5   P. S. Cameron, 'Learning with a curve: Young women's "depression" as transformative learning', V. C. X. Wang (ed.), *Handbook of Research on Adult and Community Health Education: Tools, Trends, and Methodologies* (Medical Information Science Reference/IGI Global, 2014), pp. 100–22.

Some zines are very Mad. Spandler, who has worked on a project called 'Madzines'[6] alongside *Asylum*, tells me: 'Some zines might fall apart as you open them, or the stitches can unravel. They're fragile, vulnerable, all of those things. Which is really important, because that's us – that's how we are.' Others defy tradition and formality. The title of a pamphlet by Charlie Zines – the word 'Sad!' repeated over 100 times – articulates the soul-destroying monotony of depression better than any clinical terminology. The zine's content is equally despairing and cyclical: 'Nothing I try to do to feel happy and normal seems to work! I literally fuck up everything!' You can find similarly taboo messages in Simo's zine *I Am Trash: a zine about self-hate*. The creator makes space for self-hatred and utter despair with no beginning, middle and end, no obligatory recovery narrative. It is uncomfortable to read, but that is also how it feels to really go through it.

In political movements, 'prefiguration'[7] describes the idea that we should infuse our present actions with the values that we would like to see in future utopias. The disability activist Leah Lakshmi Piepzna-Samarasinha describes prefiguration as: 'waking up and acting as if the revolution has happened.'[8] These actions might be big or small, experimental or methodical. Either way, they are about bringing the futures that only exist in our most distant imaginations into the present. While we might say that the political and economic conditions that would allow these worlds to be fully realised do not currently exist, prefiguration argues that we already have many of the tools and capabilities, that the world we want already exists in 'fragments

---

6   www.madzines.org (last accessed January 2023).

7   C. Boggs, 'Marxism, prefigurative communism, and the problem of workers' control', *Radical America* 11 (November 1977), p. 100.

8   L. L. Piepzna-Samarasinha, *Care work: Dreaming Disability Justice* (Vancouver: Arsenal Pulp Press, 2018).

and pieces, experiments and possibilities.'[9] The word in itself has artistic connotations, perhaps of trying to sketch out an image of a scene before it has actually happened. Spandler tells me that, in a way, zines are a form of prefigurative mental health politics.

> I've got this thing at the moment about 'being with' zines, and sort of just sitting with them, rather than trying to analyse them or make sense of them. It's interesting because this is one of the things survivors say they want from mental health services – someone to be alongside them through their distress and struggle.

By 'being with' zines, accepting the strangeness and subjectivity of art, and resisting the urge to authoritatively and impatiently diagnose it, we prefigure a different approach to mental health. Rather than trying to make experiences quickly legible and treatable, we acknowledge that they take time and space to understand. Spandler says:

> Sometimes I get zines where I sit and look at them and think, I don't fucking understand what this is about at all. It's just a blob or something. But this is the diversity of human experience. Sometimes it's pretty mad, but we need to be able to sit with it all.

Art in the asylum

As an expression of imagination, art is always swelling and pushing against the political limits of this world. It is therefore

---

9   R. W. Gilmore and L. Lambert, 'Making abolition geography in California's Central Valley with Ruth Wilson Gilmore', *Funambulist*, 21 (Jan/Feb 2019), https://thefunambulist.net/magazine/21-space-activism/interview-making-abolition-geography-california-central-valley-ruth-wilson-gilmore (last accessed January 2023).

also a tool that we can use to craft other political possibilities. In 2014, the artist and activist James Leadbitter embarked on an interdisciplinary project called 'Madlove', in which he hosted workshops with survivors and service users to reclaim the setting of the 'asylum' – choosing this word because it was once supposed to mean 'refuge' or 'sanctuary'. Returning to the core concepts of 'safety' or 'asylum', the project asked the question: 'Is it possible to go mad in a positive way? How would you create a safe place in which to do so? If you designed your own asylum, what would it be like?'[10]

After ideas were crowdsourced, consolidated and sketched out, most of the 'asylums' that the groups designed couldn't look more different to the setting of the psychiatric hospital. They were community-led dreams that railed against the cold, punitive nature of the ward, which is characterised by rules, rationality, restriction and seclusion. Ideas included open spaces, teleportation systems to summon up friends and family, dance floors, weather rooms, art galleries, birdhouses, swimming pools, rocket ships, and rooms where you are allowed to smash things up or throw paint. Some people resisted the idea that it needed to be a distinct place at all, saying: 'the hospital I need to be in is my flat – but made safe'.[11]

This type of imagining, far beyond the bounds of 'rational thought', is unmistakably Mad. But it is also revolutionary, forcing us to think beyond the misery and limitation of the punishing capitalist world we have come to know. The link between these two worlds – the impossible and the possible – is imagi-

---

10   http://thevacuumcleaner.co.uk/madlove-a-designer-asylum/ (last accessed January 2023).

11   https://slate.com/human-interest/2015/03/madlove-a-designer-asylum-from-james-leadbitter-the-vacuum-cleaner-is-a-mental-health-space-designed-by-patients-in-the-u-k.html (last accessed January 2023).

nation. In its most childlike and optimistic form, we are able to transcend the rigid constraints of our constructed reality, and grasp towards the world we desire. It is this belief that we can, that we must strive towards things that others say are impossible, that we must hold on to. Even the most fantastical ideas that came out of Madlove point towards fundamental desires that the hospital deprives people of: access to nature, art, music, literature, community, autonomy, pleasure, play, abundance, individuality and freedom from coercion.

Later in 2014, Leadbitter and others used ideas from the workshops to build an exhibit in Liverpool, which pointed towards many of the same desires. Some of the installations bore a physical resemblance to features of psychiatric detention today, for example, a room that repurposed the idea of the padded cell. However, its use and intention was transformed; it resembled a pillow fort that people could *choose* to go in if they wanted to cool off in privacy, to which they held the key. Another part of the exhibit featured a set of steps that you could climb to gain a bird's eye view of the space. This reflected the common desire to retreat 'up high',[12] and to gain spatial autonomy and control – the opposite of being restrained on the floor of a ward.

Art is not 'productive' or 'practical' in the way we might want it to be. It doesn't provide us with the certainty of absolute knowledge that we so often desire – there is no one interpretation or direction. But this is what makes art a Mad and liberatory tool. It demands that we dream more wildly, and shatter the Western expectations of form, tradition and categorisation, and we cannot afford not to. This venture is never individual, always political. Art demands to be seen, interpreted and responded to,

---

12   https://www.bbc.co.uk/news/av/health-32035911 (last accessed January 2023).

rupturing the confines of the lab experiment, the doctor's office, the therapy room or the bare walls of the psychiatric ward.

In 2020, Bethlem Hospital in South London hosted an installation by artist Mark Titchner at the boundary of the site – the line between psychiatric detention and the 'free' world. The artwork was made up of placards, which had questions relating to capacity and detention printed on them, for example: 'ARE YOU FREE TO DETERMINE YOUR OWN ACTIONS?'[13] One night, in the midst of the global Black Lives Matter uprisings, someone graffitied over the placards in red spray paint. The text, which was discovered in the morning, read: 'RIP SENI' – a tribute to Seni Lewis, who had been restrained at Bethlem a decade prior, leading to his death. It evoked a history that the institution had obscured from view – but art had emerged from the fringes, imploring us to look, imploring us to remember.

---

13   https://bethlemgallery.com/whats-on/some-questions-about-us (last accessed January 2023).

Chapter 9

Law and disorder

This chapter contains discussions of police violence, psychiatric abuse, sexual assault, self-harm and suicide.

Seni Lewis was 23 years old when he was restrained by 11 police officers on the floor of a padded cell, leading to his death. Described by his mother Aji as a 'gentle giant', Lewis had been admitted to Bethlem Hospital in 2010, after a drug had left him feeling agitated and strange. When Lewis' mental health crisis began, Aji had thought that a psychiatric hospital would be a place of safety and care for her son.

Later that evening, Lewis was brutalised by police. A hospital worker had called them to the ward after Lewis had allegedly damaged a door, and when they arrived, 11 officers restrained him for 40 minutes. Despite Lewis crying that he couldn't breathe, the police ignored his pleas. Lewis eventually suffered from brain stem death, and was transferred to intensive care within two hours of having been dropped off at Bethlem. He died days later.

In recent years, the public has turned its attention to the violence of policing and prisons. The Black Lives Matter movement, alongside numerous reports of police brutality, sexual assault and other abuses of power, have shed light on the harms of state systems that work together to incarcerate people (also known as 'carceral' systems). There is also a growing understanding that these systems primarily serve to control and punish poor and racialised communities, who are disproportionately policed and imprisoned. However, it is crucial to acknowledge that these systems also disproportionately punish Mad/Mentally Ill people, and share substantial practical and logical overlap with the mental health system.

Policing and mental health

Black men are particularly likely to be brutalised by the police during a mental health crisis. In 1999, a Black man called Roger Sylvester died from brain damage and cardiac arrest after being detained under the Mental Health Act and restrained by eight police officers.[1] His neighbours had called the police.[2] In 2001, a Black man named Mikey Powell died after the police hit him with a car, sprayed him with tear gas and restrained him during a mental health episode.[3] His distraught mother had called the police for help.[4] In 2008, Sean Rigg, who had a diagnosis of paranoid schizophrenia, was handcuffed and restrained by police for eight minutes during a mental health crisis, leading to his death.[5] As his body lay lifeless on the floor of Brixton Police Station, one officer accused him of 'faking it' – the same allegation levelled at Seni Lewis when he went limp after being restrained. In each of these situations, Black people's distress has been met with a combination of punishment and neglect.

---

1   https://theguardian.com/uk/2003/oct/03/ukcrime.prisonsandprobation (last accessed January 2023).

2   Ibid.

3   https://inquest.org.uk/blog/a-legacy-for-mikey-powell (last accessed January 2023).

4   Ibid.

5   https://4frontproject.org/sean-rigg (last accessed January 2023).

These cases speak to police racism, but they also demonstrate the state violence directed towards Mad/Mentally Ill people. Over a five-year period, over half of deaths in or following police contact in England and Wales were people who had 'mental health concerns'. Many of the names that ring out at protests – Dalian Atkinson, Leon Briggs, Kingsley Burrell, Kevin Clarke and Darren Cumberbatch – are those who found themselves at the crossroads of state racism *and* sanism. These two forces work together to produce particularly violent outcomes for Black people who are not seen to be sane. Signs of distress, or a lack of conformity to behavioural norms, are readily viewed through the lens of violence and criminality rather than vulnerability. We see the impact of this in the disproportionate number of Black people detained under the Mental Health Act,[6] and who are deemed to be 'a risk to themselves or others'. Black people are also 40% more likely to make contact with mental health services through the police or criminal justice system[7] – society recognises their danger before it recognises their distress.

The management and control of Mad/Mentally Ill people has also long been baked into the function of policing. Before 1961, people could be arrested and sent to prison for attempting to take their own lives – a legacy that lives on the colloquial term 'committing suicide'. Today, the Mental Health Act provides the police with emergency powers to enter a person's home and take them to a 'place of safety' (until recent years, usually a police cell) under section 135 and 136. It is estimated that up to 40% of police time is spent responding to incidents that are linked

6   https://ethnicity-facts-figures.service.gov.uk/health/mental-health/detentions-under-the-mental-health-act/latest (last accessed January 2023).

7   https://mind.org.uk/news-campaigns/legal-news/legal-newsletter-june-2019/discrimination-in-mental-health-services (last accessed January 2023).

to mental health.[8] As the institution deployed to manage populations that are disruptive to capital accumulation and societal 'order', it should be no surprise that police play a key role in mental health crisis response. The punishment, incarceration and violence enacted on Mad/Mentally Ill people by police is not a side effect of policing, but the intended outcome.

More recently, police have also served a function in gatekeeping mental health resources from those whose rehabilitation into the workforce is deemed too costly or impossible. In 2021, the 'Stop SIM' campaign drew attention to the ways that the police collaborates with the NHS in denying people support. The campaign resisted the 'Serenity Integrated Mentoring' (SIM) model of care, which was introduced by NHS England and uses police as part of community mental health teams and crisis care. The model, which at the time of writing is used in almost half of England's NHS trusts, instructs emergency services not to treat people who are very unwell and frequently come into contact with them. One of the architects of the SIM model described the behaviours of these people as 'attention-seeking', and argued that they place an 'unnecessary financial burden' on the NHS.[9] Within the model, police officers are also contracted by the NHS to coerce these people into no longer contacting emergency services. This serves the function of ring-fencing state resources for those whose recovery is seen to be a viable and lucrative investment.

The SIM model is far from a novel development. Rather, it draws attention to the continued collaboration and blurring of

---

8 https://theguardian.com/uk-news/2016/jan/27/mental-health-crisis-huge-increasing-share-police-time-40 (last accessed January 2023).

9 P. Jennings and C. B. Matheson-Monnet, 'Multi-agency mentoring pilot intervention for high intensity service users of emergency public services: the Isle of Wight Integrated Recovery Programme', *Journal of Criminological Research, Policy and Practice*, 3:2, (2017), pp. 105–18.

boundaries between health services and the police. In Britain, the police are deployed to respond to people in crisis; cross the threshold into services; help restrain and detain people; and, within the SIM model and counterterrorism strategies like Prevent, can gain access to people's medical records. Our 'health' is always at service to the state, and police involvement in mental health services reminds us of this. The effect of this is that 'care' becomes inseparable from punishment and neglect. Rizwaan Sabir, a British Muslim who was falsely arrested in 2008 under the Prevent strategy, tells me that he avoided going to mental health services during a crisis because he was afraid of record-sharing between the NHS and the police. In a statement that speaks to the broader overlap between institutions, Sabir says: 'In my mind at that time, there was no difference between a police officer and a doctor.'

Prisons and mental health

Just beyond the horizon of policing lurks the prison – a physical space that contains and disciplines large numbers of Mad/ Mentally Ill people. It is estimated that up to 90% of prisoners in England and Wales are in some way mentally unwell. The causes of this statistic are plural, since prisons actively produce distress, but they are also a state response to illness and suffering that is created by our societal conditions. According to research from 1998, 22% of women remand prisoners in England and Wales have previously been admitted to a psychiatric hospital.[10] Meanwhile, 84% of men in prison have had an adverse childhood experience like exposure to abuse, alcoholism, drug use or

---

10   N. Singleton, H. Meltzer and R. Gatward, 'Psychiatric Morbidity among Prisoners in England and Wales', Office for National Statistics, (London: Stationery Office, 1998).

domestic violence at home.[11] However, the prison environment that these people enter into is undoubtedly one where they will be further punished and traumatised.

Christina*, who was arrested during a mental health crisis, tells me about her daily schedule when she was in prison. 'You're locked in your cell, come out for a meal, locked in your cell, come out for a meal . . . it's very, very monotonous. It's not a therapeutic environment.' When they were short-staffed, coming out of her cell wasn't even a possibility, and Christina might be trapped in the space for up to 24 hours a day. She tells me that, particularly as she was staying on a mental health unit of the prison, she was enclosed in a claustrophobic space with lots of people who were unwell. Prisons do not only extract people's time, they also systematically extract people's health and well-being, because the state is less concerned with maintaining prisoner health for the purposes of exploitation. Many Mad/Mentally Ill prisoners are unable to gain access to medication in prison – for example, Sarah Reed, who took her own life in prison in 2016 after being denied access to psychiatric medication. Between 2021–2, there were 70 self-inflicted deaths and almost 53,000 self-harm incidents in English and Welsh prisons.[12] Poor well-being is not a side effect, but a core function of the prison – which systematically neglects supposedly 'disorderly' and 'unproductive' people's needs, allowing them to suffer, get sick and die. Here we can see a link to the emergence of the asylums in the nineteenth century, and their role in warehousing people who could not be exploited on the production line.

---

11   https://itv.com/news/wales/2019-04-29/more-than-eight-in-ten-men-in-prison-suffered-childhood-adversity-new-report (last accessed January 2023).

* Name has been changed.

12   https://gov.uk/government/statistics/safety-in-custody-quarterly-update-to-june-2022/safety-in-custody-statistics-england-and-wales-deaths-in-prison-custody-to-september-2022-assaults-and-self-harm-to-june-2022 (last accessed January 2023).

The mental distress wrought on prisoners can't be understood on an individual basis. The after-effects of punishment and seclusion don't only live on for prisoners themselves – they are also held in the bodyminds of loved ones, and ripple across communities and generations. It is estimated that 15% of prisoners' children meet the criteria for post traumatic stress disorder (PTSD),[13] with some people reporting flashbacks of their loved ones being taken away by the police.[14] The impacts of imprisonment therefore cannot be contained within the cell or the institution – it creates suffering on a broader social level, which also creates more potential prisoners.

When we think of institutions that are bound up with mental health, we often think of medicine, psychology and psychiatry. However, the line between the constructed categories of 'criminal' and 'Mad/Mentally Ill' is by no means clear cut, and there are many things shared between them. The state sorts each group into these categories because of their failure to 'behave' as pliable or exploitable citizens. In each case, their disorderliness is also overwhelmingly the result of their social and economic circumstances. As a result, both groups are disciplined by the same violent systems, which ultimately produce more distress and 'disorder'.

'Care' and carcerality

It is also important to connect the dots between punishment and incarceration (or 'carcerality') and the mental health system itself. One clear example of carcerality in the mental health

---

13   G. Gualtieri, F. Ferretti, A. Masti, A. Pozza and A. Coluccia, 'Post-traumatic Stress Disorder in prisoners' offspring: A systematic review and meta-analysis', *Clinical Practice and Epidemiology in Mental Health*, 16, (Apr 2020), pp. 36–45.

14   https://initiatejustice.org/transcript-season-1-episode-7-disability-justice/ (last accessed January 2023).

system is detention under the Mental Health Act, which is used to override the autonomy of Mad/Mentally Ill people and institutionalise them. As discussed in Chapter 1, state detention was not always the default approach, but a development that responded to the capitalist system. Those who could not be exploited, controlled or cared for in this new society needed somewhere to go. Today, detentions mirror the racialised patterns seen in policing and imprisonment; as earlier discussed, Black people are almost five times as likely to be detained under the Mental Health Act than their white counterparts. The act is also responsible for the largest proportion of all deaths in state custody in England and Wales – at 60%.[15] Further research has found that people are at an increased risk of dying after state detention.[16,17]

Similarly to the prison system, psychiatric detention separates people from the 'outside world', even if they have loved ones who can provide them with care and support. When people are compulsorily detained, they are removed from their communities and placed in settings with lots of other powerless and distressed people, sometimes in units that are far from home. Entering detention is not a choice, and leaving it is not a choice either; decisions regarding release rest with a healthcare professional, rather than with the person themselves. As a result, people may be detained for years with no idea of when they will

15   www.inquest.org.uk/deaths-in-mental-health-detention (last accessed January 2023).

16   R. Musgrove, M. Carr, N. Kapur, C. Chew-Graham, F. Mughal, D. Ashcroft and R. Webb, 'Suicide and other causes of death among working-age and older adults in the year after discharge from in-patient mental healthcare in England: Matched cohort study', *British Journal of Psychiatry*, 221:2, (2022), pp. 468–75.

17   D. Osborn, G. Favarato, D. Lamb, T. Harper, S. Johnson, B. Lloyd-Evans and S. Weich, 'Readmission after discharge from acute mental healthcare among 231 988 people in England: Cohort study exploring predictors of readmission including availability of acute day units in local areas', *BJPsych Open*, 7(4):e136, (July 2021).

be released – particularly autistic and learning-disabled people, for whom the average length of hospital stay is 5.4 years, and over 50% of which are detained for over two years.[18] In 2021 and 2022, two British autistic men were released from hospital after 15 and 21 years respectively.[19] Even those who have short stays often get stuck in a revolving door, with more than one in five patients being readmitted within six months of release from acute psychiatric inpatient stay.[20] This challenges the idea that long-term institutionalisation is a relic of the past; for some, it essentially continues under a different guise.

Restraint plays a prominent role in policing, prisons and mental health systems. Alongside Seni Lewis, there have been many other restraint-related injuries and deaths in the mental health system. In 1998, David 'Rocky' Bennett died after being restrained for around 25 minutes on a psychiatric unit in Norwich.[21] Unlike Lewis, Bennett wasn't restrained by police, but rather by five NHS nurses. Data collected between 2011–12 found that over the course of one year, there were over 1,000 incidents of physical injury in English mental health services, and 3,000 instances of face-down restraint[22] (which is considered the most dangerous form). It is not uncommon for people to be left with friction burns, bruises or even broken bones after

18   https://digital.nhs.uk/data-and-information/publications/statistical/learning-disability-services-statistics/at-november-2021-mhsds-september-2021-final/ (last accessed January 2023).

19   https://bbc.co.uk/news/uk-62819017 (last accessed January 2023).

20   Osborn, et al., 'Readmission after discharge from acute mental healthcare among 231 988 people in England'.

21   https://www.theguardian.com/uk/2004/feb/06/race.politics   (last   accessed January 2023).

22   https://mind.org.uk/media-a/4378/physical_restraint_final_web_version.pdf (last accessed January 2023).

being restrained. Meanwhile, Black people are more likely to be restrained on wards than white people.[23]

Restraint isn't only mechanical; it can also be chemical, for example being forcibly injected with drugs or made to swallow medication; or through seclusion, like being locked in a padded cell. Each of these practices are forms of curative violence, which prioritise a particular vision of 'health' over the person's needs and desires. Their primary aim is also to create docility in institutional settings. Writer and researcher Oliver* tells me of his lasting trauma after being restrained, and possibly forcibly injected, under section:

> [The nurses] were observing me through glass, and some of them were laughing at me. When they came in to give me medication, they made me put my hands up and lay down, and there were literally 10 people pinning me down. I think I even got injected with something. After that incident, I just kept having flashbacks to that time. You're treated like an animal – honestly, there's no other way to describe it.

Restraint is a form of suppression, so we should ask: what does suppression *do*? When the police suppress working class protest, when prisons suppress racialised communities, when people are socialised to suppress their emotions, particularly in the face of injustice? Suppression attempts to quash 'disorder' or resistance, often amplifying it in either the short or long term. It tries to make disorderliness or dissent disappear without listening to it, or remedying its origins. When states suppress people, they frequently find that no tool will seem to ever be powerful enough

---

23   https://mind.org.uk/news-campaigns/legal-news/legal-newsletter-june-2019/
discrimination-in-mental-health-services/ (last accessed January 2023).

* Name has been changed.

– from weapons, to censorship, to surveillance – and so suppression techniques become increasingly elaborate, invasive and severe.

Parallel to an experience of prisons, Mad/Mentally Ill people often find themselves closely surveilled on psychiatric wards. Christina, who was transferred to a psychiatric ward after being in prison, tells me that she was often put on 'level three' observation on the ward, in which 'a staff member is looking at you constantly, even when you go to the toilet and have a shower. That was really humiliating . . . it made me want to self-harm even more.' In 2021, 23 NHS trusts also came under fire for their use of Oxevision, a monitoring system that allowed them to film psychiatric patients in their bedrooms without their knowledge or consent.[24] Here, we can see a parallel to the expansion of all kinds of surveillance under neoliberalism, for example, the Prevent strategy, which aims to identify and punish 'extremist' behaviours.[25] In both cases, increasing state intrusion and control of 'disorderly' behaviour is justified under the guise of 'care' and 'safety' for its citizens.

The logics of incarceration are also weaved into the most everyday realities of psychiatric detention. Similarly to the era of moral treatment, people's activities and schedules are closely controlled; and professionals are able to control people's access to food, privacy, the outside world, contact with others, phones and various other 'contraband' items. This suppression often ultimately leads to greater distress. Oliver uses the word

---

24   https://theguardian.com/society/2021/dec/13/nhs-trusts-urged-to-ditch-oxevision-system-covert-surveillance-mental-health-patients (last accessed January 2023).

25   I. Zempi and A. Tripli, 'Listening to Muslim students' voices on the Prevent duty in British universities: A qualitative study', *Education, Citizenship and Social Justice*, 0:0, (2022).

'punished', saying: 'I kept protesting, I kept saying that I wanted to be released . . . I really hated it. It was probably one of the worst experiences I've ever had.' Christina echoes these sentiments, saying that when she was admitted without leave to a 'secure unit' (mental health units that predominantly detain people who have been arrested or imprisoned), she was entirely at the mercy of professionals: 'I was completely confined to the hospital, and the doctors had the sole power to decide when you can start your leave, how long you can go out for, and who you can go with. You have no power whatsoever . . . it was like being in prison again.'

This lack of power means that a person's rights and 'privileges' on the ward, as well as their ability to be released, become dependent on what professionals perceive to be 'good' behaviour. This also often implicitly encourages Mad/Mentally Ill people to suppress their feelings in order to 'succeed' by the rules of the ward. Here, we see an echo of the dissociation and alienation that we have already discussed as part of the rules of the education system and the workplace under capitalism. In all of these spaces, our survival and 'autonomy' is dependent on splitting off from our true emotions and maintaining a mask.

As well as using similar mechanisms and logics, the prison and mental health systems often directly collaborate with one another in their mutual quest for human 'correction'.[26] For example, the psychiatric diagnosis of anti-social personality disorder (ASPD, still commonly referred to as 'psychopathy') uses 'criminal behaviour' as part of its diagnostic criteria, and helps prop up the idea that some people need to be incarcerated

---

26   L. Ben-Moshe, *Decarcerating Disability: Deinstitutionalization and Prison Abolition* (Minneapolis: University of Minnesota Press, 2020).

for life.[27] On an institutional level, 'maximum security' psychiatric facilities like Berkshire's Broadmoor Hospital admit people through prisons and courts, and have come under fire in recent decades for allegedly implementing razor-wire fences and using arm and leg shackles for restraint.[28] At Broadmoor, the average length of stay is five and a half years,[29] however in 2003, the facility released a 94-year-old woman who had been detained for 40 years[30] – essentially a life sentence.

The harms of the mental health system are not neatly contained within the walls of psychiatric facilities – they spill out into the world beyond them too. As mentioned in Chapter 1, detention is also a deterrent, as it reminds people of the grave potential consequences of nonconformity. Few people are entirely comfortable with the idea of being sectioned, regardless of how much we know about what it is like to be detained. This can and is used against us. For example, Oliver says that, after his section ended, the lingering possibility of being detained again was used against him during subsequent mental health treatment. 'I was told that if I didn't take the medication, I was going to be sectioned again . . . [but when I was medicated] I constantly felt like a zombie, and couldn't do basic things.' Liat Ben-Moshe has described this phenomenon as 'the institution to come'[31] – a threat that hangs over all of our heads as we move

---

27 Defences of the prison and the psychiatric ward both often hinge on the call: 'but what about the psychopaths, rapists and murderers?'

28 https://theguardian.com/society/2002/jul/17/mentalhealth.guardian societysupplement (last accessed January 2023).

29 https://westlondon.nhs.uk/our-services/adult/secure-services/broadmoor-hospital (last accessed January 2023).

30 https://theguardian.com/uk/2003/dec/10/health.mentalhealth (last accessed January 2023).

31 Ben-Moshe, *Decarcerating Disability*.

through the world, quietly reminding us that we must be (or at least appear) sane.

This phenomenon impacts on the honesty of our interactions with doctors, psychologists and therapists in particular – as the threat of section is always a silent participant in the room. It means that people in distress may actively avoid discussing suicidal thoughts with professionals, out of fear that they will be sectioned if they are deemed, according to professionals' subjective judgement, to be 'at risk'. Even if we are not always conscious of it, the appearance of sanity is also necessary in public spaces, since anyone has the ability to call the police on someone who exhibits what they personally deem to be 'strange behaviour'. Therefore the *fear* of punishment, including material consequences like having children taken away, prevents us from being honest, getting support, or even just being ourselves in daily life. It transforms mental 'health' into something we have no choice but to practise and perform – a logic that spills out further into neoliberal messaging that we all *must* look after ourselves and maintain our bodyminds in line with the demands of the state.

While many people with traumatising past experiences work to minimise contact with the mental health system, we should also remember that others want to access resources that are gatekept within it. As earlier discussed, within the SIM model, people may find themselves barred from services for being the 'wrong kind of sick'. Others, who are deemed to be 'not sick enough', may find themselves neglected on waiting lists until they are in crisis, at which point they may be sectioned and treated punitively. However, these are not different or contradictory issues. Both abuse and neglect ultimately stem from the control exerted over Mad/Mentally Ill people, in a system in which they do not have a real say in their care.

There is a long history of agitation and organising against the carceral nature of state mental health systems. In the 1970s, the US Black Panthers intuitively made links between asylums and prisons because members had frequently been incarcerated in mental hospitals.[32] When London's Mental Patients' Union was formed during the same decade, members produced a pamphlet calling for the abolition of compulsory hospitalisation and compulsory treatment.[33] However, the current climate of NHS cuts and years-long waiting lists has stifled our ability to imagine boldly towards more liberating forms of 'mental healthcare'. While many of us argue for more funding and expansion in a struggle to access resources, this is an apt moment to interrogate what kinds of mental healthcare we want. Do we want a system that shuts people in and shuts people out? A system whose structures are focused on managing us in line with economic demands, rather than honouring our individuality and helping us heal? Are capitalist neoliberal 'services' the best we can dream of?

Transforming the world

I want to call on our imaginations to interrogate the idea that these systems still broadly 'work' for many. Does calling the police in crisis situations 'work' when it might result in death? Does restraint 'work', when it destroys trust, and traumatises and kills people? Does the mental health system 'work' when we are at the constant mercy of professionals, and will never be on equal footing? Does institutionalisation 'work' when people are

---

32 S. Schalk, *Black Disability Politics* (Durham, NC: Duke University Press, 2022).
33 https://libcom.org/article/mental-patients-union-1973 (last accessed January 2023).

removed from their families for years? When we all navigate the system under the threat of section, abuse or neglect?

Following the Black Lives Matter uprisings of 2020, the work of Black feminist activist scholars like Angela Davis and Ruth Wilson Gilmore has grown in popularity, alongside the resurgence of an 'abolitionist' movement. Abolition feminism, specifically, is a liberatory vision for the organisation of social life free from all forms of violence. It necessitates an end to carceral logics and all forms of imprisonment, surveillance, counterterror, policing, punishment and exile.[34] Public discourses are hostile to abolitionist politics, which are often framed as 'loony' or actively dangerous. However, the politics of abolition *seeks* to be bold, transformative and revolutionary. It threatens everything we have learned about how the world works. Abolition does not only work towards a world without incarceration, but one that deconstructs the logics, practices, economic realities and desires that make incarceration possible in the first place. It sees 'abolition' not only as an event, but an intentional, long-term vision for structuring our entire society, and of thinking and relating to one another.

Abolitionists demand that we move away from punishment and harm in all arenas of our lives: policing, prisons, education, borders, medicine, our relationships, our families, our communities and the ways that we think about ourselves. Abolitionists point out that the spectre of policing is everywhere – when children are excluded from school, when we are encouraged to report 'suspicious' people to authorities, when people can't access healthcare because of their BMI or migration status. Abolitionists across each of these arenas also share an understanding

---

34 https://bcrw.barnard.edu/event/abolition-feminism-celebrating-20-years-of-incite/ (last accessed January 2023).

that the state and its institutions ultimately do not keep us safe,[35] even if we must engage with them in practice. However, during the widespread protest of 2020, I saw many people stating that funding should simply be redirected from policing to state mental health systems. This overlooks the fact that, for many people, the mental health system currently functions as a site of policing, punishment and incarceration. Police help detain and restrain in the system, but more broadly, the logics of seclusion, coercion, force, and punishment are baked into the power dynamics of the system. Therefore we need to extend abolitionist politics to the mental health system too.

Abolishing all carceral approaches to mental health sounds unthinkable to many – including many people who engage with these systems to stay alive. Since the days of the asylum, it has been taken for granted that Mad/Mentally Ill people are dangerous to themselves and others, and that there is no alternative but to lock them up, restrain them and 'treat' them against their will. But we should flip this totalising statement on its head and grasp towards the opposite assumption – that it is *always possible* to find an alternative. What transformation would occur if we centred harm reduction, de-escalation, compassion and community, and tried every possible alternative we could think of before violating someone's bodily autonomy? What if these principles were embedded in both our relations, and in larger systems and structures divorced from the state?

Picture the scenario that you are afraid of – the person who is 'too Mad' or violent or suicidal to be cared for or reasoned with. What happened to them? What do they need to feel better? Why are they doing what they're doing? If they are confused or angry, what might calm them? If you were in their situation, how

---

35   A. Day and S. McBean, *Abolition Revolution* (London: Pluto Press, 2022).

would you feel? What alternative is there to calling the police? If you feel you can't communicate with them, or they aren't in a place to direct their own care or treatment, have you tried every option? Who might know them well and could help guide the path forward? What medications, people, places or practices has the person previously said that they would want in a crisis situation like this? If we imagine a Black person who is in distress, or is perceived to be behaving aggressively because they are scared – the introduction of police into the situation will most likely make their fear and distress worse. They might run away or hide, because they have learned that it is not okay to show signs of crisis. Alternately, we could call other loved ones, who might know what the person needs. We could try to understand the sources triggering these emotions and remove them. We could focus on the safety of the person as well as ourselves.

This is not to downplay the seriousness of mental health crises. Many people do want plans in place to make sure they stay inside when a crisis comes on, or want a place to go away from other people to minimise harm or gain respite. But the reality is that most people are not offered anything other than the current system.

Disability justice starts from the principle that everyone has the right to a life in the community. It opposes psychiatric incarceration and segregation as the answer to complex social problems, and doesn't see personhood and autonomy as conditional on how able-bodied/minded a person appears to be. It sees care as centred around trust, not trickery or coercion. It asks us to interrogate which elements people need, and challenges us to reimagine them in safe, well-resourced and accountable community spaces. This is what we should be striving towards as we resist carcerality in all its forms.

Transformative justice is an approach that aims to respond to harm without creating more harm. It asks that we do not individualise harm, but address the *causes* of harm, which are wide-ranging and systemic. This is a logic that we must extend to mental health, and, in particular, mental health crisis. Self-harm and suicide are often responses to feeling trapped and powerless. Therefore framing self-harm as a purely personal risk freezes harm in the present, never getting to the root of where it came from.

A transformative justice approach for mental health means creating a world where no one could get to the point of being disappeared by the state in order to stay alive. The diverse range of experiences that we call 'mental health crises' rarely spring up from nowhere. Like much of the prison population, many people in psychiatric detention have histories of abuse, deprivation, homelessness, unemployment and substance addiction.[36] If we really want them to be well, why don't we go deeper than the 'symptoms' and address the economic and relational circumstances that lead to the suffering of so many? If we turn back the clock from the moment of crisis, we can almost always find numerous moments at which a person should have received care or attention, but didn't have access to it. This includes the people on waiting lists, but it also means those without adequate living and working conditions; financial security; safety from violence; freedom from oppression; community; love; creativity; autonomy. When we look at these things – at all the ways we could prevent crises in the first place – it is clear that the punishment of Mad/Mentally Ill people is not inevitable. Abolition is often framed as chaos and disorder, but abolitionist politics show us that our current reality is chaotic and disorderly.

---

36 L. Birmingham, 'Mental disorder and prisons', *Psychiatric Bulletin*, 28:11, (2004), pp. 393–7.

Ruth Wilson Gilmore says: 'abolition is about presence, not absence. It's about building life-affirming institutions.' If we want to end incarceration in all its forms, we need to build a world where we do not reactively force people to live, but one that is survivable. Like revolutionary abolitionists, I do not see this as a simple policy proposal – I believe it demands creative imagination, and the transformation of the entire fabric of our society. This is an intentionally threatening and terrifying vision, which is not restricted to any one specific locale. The outcomes of deinstitutionalisation in the twentieth century show us that to ensure Mad/Mentally Ill people are neither abused or neglected,[37] we need to protect one another from the forces of neoliberal capitalism, racism and poverty. Then we need to overthrow them. We also need to build a world made up of strong communities, in which everyone has a network of skilled-up people to help keep themselves and others safe. Everyone must have free access to therapeutic practices and medication, without professional gatekeeping. We must be prepared for the possibility that anyone could become unwell – making sure everyone creates a support plan for what they would like to happen in a crisis. Mental health responses must be community and patient-run, well-funded, free from entrenched power dynamics, and should centre care rather than force. This would enable people to express what they want and need when they are struggling, free from the fear that they will have their autonomy or dignity violated. Although achieving this is no straightforward task, we must imagine that there is something out there better than this; and that we have the tools to create it.

---

37 H. Spandler, 'From Psychiatric Abuse to Psychiatric Neglect?' *Asylum*, 23.2, (Summer 2016), pp. 7–8.

Chapter 10

Other possibilities

So much of the work of oppression is about policing the imagination. – Saidiya Hartman

I can't tell you 100% what that future is going to look like. I can tell you what some of those pieces are going to look like, or particularly what I'm trying to create. But it's not just about me, and if you want to see what I can do, give me money and I'll do it. – Stefanie Lyn Kaufman-Mthimkhulu

They asked me, 'Where are you going with this?' and I said, 'I don't know.' And it was true. I didn't know. – Franco Basaglia

This chapter contains descriptions of self-harm and discussions of suicide.

In a small city in the North East of Italy, mental healthcare looks very different. Trieste – which is recognised by the World Health Organisation (WHO) as having one of the most advanced community healthcare systems in the world – has no psychiatric hospitals. Instead, it relies on a system of publicly funded community-based healthcare. Trieste's services reject the logics of restraint and forced treatment. Vincenzo Passante Spaccapietra, a former user of Trieste's mental health services, tells me that it is difficult to articulate its approach to British people, because it is so far from the system we are accustomed to.

> The many benefits of the system in Trieste did not strike me as surprising, but they probably would to many British observers. Nobody ever talked to me about a diagnosis, nobody ever suggested that I should take medication, and there was no waiting list to have access to psychological help. I'm sure that if I wanted to be talked to about a diagnosis, or if I wanted to take medication, that would not have been a problem.

Fundamental to the 'Trieste model' is placing the person at the centre of their mental healthcare, rather than the concept of a solely biomedical pathology. Vincenzo tells me: As part of this, the approach also centres 'wellness' – ensuring that people are as supported as they can be *before* they get to crisis point. He says: 'The goal of the system is not just to get symptoms to improve, or remain under control in a scientifically efficient way; the goal is to help the person get better, and this can rarely be achieved with pre-packaged approaches.'

For most of the twentieth century, the existence of a system like that found in Trieste would have been unthinkable. Italy, like Britain, was once populated by bleak, neglected, 'Bedlam-like' asylums in the nineteenth century, which warehoused Mad/ Mentally Ill people. During the 1960s, a common refrain among residents was that the only way people could leave the institution was 'in a coffin'.[1] However, when the left-wing Italian psychiatrist Franco Basaglia took on the role of asylum director at Trieste's San Giovanni Hospital in 1971, at the peak of the anti-psychiatry movement, he quickly acted to close the hospital

---

1 J. Foot, *The Man Who Closed the Asylums: Franco Basaglia and the Revolution in Mental Health Care*, (London and New York: Verso, 2015).

down, with patients even helping to knock down its fences and walls.[2] Basaglia had been imprisoned himself for his anti-fascist activities during the Second World War, and quickly identified the asylums he worked in as 'total institutions', which closely resembled prisons in their structures and processes. Basaglia is now the best-known figurehead of a broader Italian 'Psichiatria Democratica' (Democratic Psychiatry) movement, which sought to challenge the ideas, values and practices of traditional psychiatry. In 1978, 'Basaglia's Law' was passed, mandating that all of Italy's asylums be closed. Today, Italy is the only nation in the world to have outlawed psychiatric hospitals.

Trieste has four mental health centres, some of which look just like houses integrated on residential streets in the community. San Giovanni asylum has been converted into their offices, and painted on the side of the building is the slogan 'freedom is therapeutic'. Following this ethos, the system has a 'no locked doors' policy – all engagement with services is voluntary, and doesn't entail people being cut off from their communities. For example, service users who want to stay overnight are welcome to bring family or pets with them. There is one small 'psychiatric emergency' ward in the city, with only six beds (despite a population of just over 200,000 people). The system is, however, accessible – its doors are also open to anyone, with service users being able to simply walk in without a referral. Barcola Community Mental Health Centre in Trieste is open from 8am until 8pm, with a staff member on duty at all hours to respond to people in crisis in the night or early morning.

Their staff do not wear uniforms or name badges – relics of institutions that prop up power binaries like doctor/patient or sane/Mad. Visiting Barcola in early 2020, journalist Rob Waters

2   Ibid.

wrote: 'The center has the casual feel of a recreation center, and [service users] come and go as they wish, dropping in to have lunch, chat with friends, meet with therapists, get medication, or simply hang out.'

The Trieste model challenges the 'inevitability' of carceral approaches to mental health. Trieste is, importantly, not a utopia. The model is not equipped to challenge the broader social and economic forces that lead many of us to be distressed in the first place. Within services, there are also difficult situations, and on rare occasions people are detained for very brief periods of time. However, Passante tells me that boundaries in the system are defined 'dialectically', through long periods of negotiation and sometimes compromise. This approach is a slow one, it requires relationships characterised by trust and collaboration, rather than domination and control. One staff member told Waters:

If you can't seclude, if you can't restrain, you have to find alternatives. Maybe you go outside, go for a walk, have a coffee. If the institution is so hard, with a lot of rules and distance and locked doors, it increases the risk of violence because the institution itself is being really violent.

We are often led to believe that our societal approach to mental health, driven by capitalist qualities of impatience and rigidity, is the only way. However, when we expand our imaginations and open up space for ambiguity, collaboration, creativity, plurality and strangeness, new and surprising possibilities emerge. There is *no one way*, no perfect model or approach, but when we look hard enough at both the past and the present, we can find other glimmers of potential radical futures. Scattered across time and space, we should attempt to assemble them and learn from them.

A different approach to crisis

Survivors, service users and other Mad/Mentally Ill people have pursued the project of non-medical 'crisis houses' for decades. When the Socialist Patients' Collective (SPK) occupied the university where they conducted their organising in the 1970s, one of their demands was a residence to use as a crisis or refuge house. The same decade, Hackney Mental Patients' Union hosted people who were in crisis in the house they occupied.[3] Today, a handful of more formalised crisis houses operate across the country, functioning as alternatives to hospital admission, detainment or coercion. Some are now linked to the NHS, others operate independently. In stark contrast to the sterile psychiatric ward, these spaces emphasise a home-like environment, and usually have a small number of beds for voluntary overnight stay. Much like centres in Trieste, crisis houses are often part of residential streets, like Drayton Park Women's Crisis House in London. Unlike psychiatric wards, some crisis houses, like Link House in Bristol, give guests the option to put objects that could be used to self-injure in a box in their bedroom, which they hold the keys to. Guests also have the choice to give the keys to staff, with the option of having a conversation with staff members about their feelings before choosing whether to access the keys. Former Link House guest, Jennifer Reese, has written:

> This put me in control of my own body again. In hospital I was stealing scissors from the art room to hurt myself, hitting my head on the walls . . . At Link House I kept the keys to the

---

3 https://hackneyhistory.wordpress.com/2016/12/27/hackney-peoples-press-1975-hackney-mental-patients-union/ (last accessed January 2023).

sharps box myself. In the two weeks I was there I had access to glass and kitchen knives, and I didn't cut myself once.[4]

Some crisis houses, like the Maytree Suicide Respite Centre, are staffed by volunteers who have lived experience of feeling suicidal or supporting someone else in crisis.

Across borders and history, there have also been various attempts at establishing 'therapeutic communities' that provide alternative spaces for people experiencing mental distress or crisis. 'Soteria houses', for example, are informed by the work of the American psychiatrist Loren Mosher in the 1970s. Mosher was partly influenced by the moral treatment of the nine-teenth century, the Freudian psychoanalysis of the following century, and also residential treatment experiments like R. D. Laing's, and wanted to use these philosophies for people diag-nosed with schizophrenia. Core principles of the 'Soteria model' are that houses are run by non-medical staff, that treatment is consensual, that staff and residents are considered peers with communal responsibilities, that each person's subjective expe-rience of psychosis or 'altered states' is valued, and that there is little or no antipsychotic medication. Soteria houses have been established at various times across countries like the US, Swit-zerland, Germany and Hungary. In 2004, a Soteria Network was formed in Bradford, in the UK, 'promoting the development of drug-free and minimum medication therapeutic environments for people experiencing 'psychosis' or extreme states.'

Each of these projects honour the fact that 'forcible healing' is an oxymoron – by its nature, force violates consent and is anti-thetical to healing. While coercion may be 'effective' in the short

---

4   https://nsun.org.uk/psychiatric-hospital-left-me-suicidal-and-homeless-we-need-a-human-rights-based-approach-to-mental-health-care/ (last accessed January 2023).

term, it is only ever a quick fix. Frameworks like those used in Trieste, and by crisis and Soteria houses, grapple with the hard and complex work of *being with* someone through distress, learning about their life history and their way of understanding the world, and adapting based on the person's own preferences.

Community care

Following deinstitutionalisation, Margaret Thatcher's vision of 'care in the community' was never truly caring. It was driven by the desire for cost-effectiveness, and produced policies like Community Treatment Orders (CTOs), which coerce people into taking medication even outside of institutions. However, grassroots groups have consistently pioneered genuine community care. The Fireweed Collective, a US-based mental health education and mutual aid group, has devised a form of support plan called 'Mad maps'. Mad maps help people chart their own desires, dreams, and supports that they need when they are struggling, so that others can better care for them in times of mental distress. People who make Mad maps may craft their own 'wellness/safety team' of people to help them when they are in crisis. The document itself helps this group of nominated people in performing that role, and can be particularly useful in times of crisis in which the person feels they can no longer communicate their needs and desires. When people make Mad maps, prompts might include: 'what would a happy life look like?', 'in what ways can psychiatric diagnosis be helpful/unhelpful for me?', 'what are signs that I have entered a crisis?', 'what concrete things can people do to help?', 'at what point do I feel I can no longer make decisions for myself, and who do I want/not want to make decisions for me?', 'what treatments are acceptable/not acceptable?', and 'what do I want my supporters to do if I'm a danger to myself or others?' Through questions like this, Mad maps allow people to make clear what kind of care they want in advance of a crisis, helping establish and honour consent, and ensuring everyone is kept safe. Mad maps are not one-size-fits-all – they accommodate our wide-ranging relationships to our own mental states. Some people may want their wellness/safety teams to make sure they stay inside, or to help them gain access to specific medications or treatment facilities. But Mad maps first and foremost honour the autonomy of the person experiencing crisis. They resist binary conceptions of consent, which tell us that when consent becomes complicated, the state must override it entirely.

Some grassroots groups have also worked to establish their own mental health response teams, which do not involve the police in responding to extreme mental distress. The US-based collective Mental Health First aims to interrupt and eliminate the need for police involvement in mental health crisis first response. Run by volunteer community members, Mental Health First teams provide mobile peer support, de-escalation assistance, and non-punitive and life-affirming interventions for people in crisis. In Britain, Campaign for Psych Abolition (CPA), a grassroots group against psychiatry, policing and prisons, has established a guide for creating local 'Comrades Care Teams', a form of decentralised community response that anyone can set up. These teams allow comrades to put a callout to others in their local area if they are struggling and need company and support. Queercare, a UK-based transfeminist autonomous care organisation, has also established a protocol for mental health intervention, which steers away from controlling and pathologising approaches. As part of their work, they also advocate for people in contact with mental health services – usually supporting people who want to avoid being sectioned.

Community care also sometimes comes in the form of 'peer support', a practice in which people who have lived experience of mental distress support one another. People in a peer support group might share a diagnosis, or have some other shared affinity like being queer or a person of colour; and they may come together to discuss their experiences or do other kinds of communal activity. Peer support is about honouring our collective knowledge and allowing us to lead with our own expertise.

Depathologisation

Since Mad Pride sprung out of Toronto, Canada, in 1993, events under this banner have taken place at various times and across borders: in the UK, Ireland, Germany, Spain, Portugal, Brazil, Mexico, the US, South Africa and Korea. Mad Pride is a celebration for anyone who might be categorised by the world as Mad/Mentally Ill. Marches have often involved 'bed pushes', in which people push wheeled gurneys down the street. Sometimes marchers dress up like doctors and nurses, in an effort to mock and start conversations about psychiatric abuse; in other instances, beds are simply colourfully decorated, as a means of 'celebrat[ing] Mad peoples' journey from the institution to the community'.[5]

Mad Pride's logo – a person defiantly breaking free from their chains – sits alongside the slogan: 'The right to be free . . . the right to be me'. It is a radical rebuttal to psychiatric pathologisation, which frames Madness as a biomedical sickness to be cured. Inspired by gay pride protests, it also nods towards the often-erased shared history between Mad and queer people, indicating that their paths forward might be marked by similar

---

5   http://torontomadpride.com/2016/03/mad-pride-parade-bed-push/ (last accessed January 2023).

acts of public 'reclaiming' and resistance in the face of oppression. In 2022, CPA hosted the first Mad Pride event in London in over ten years, demonstrating renewed consciousness of, and appetite for, reclaiming Madness and contesting psychiatric control.

We can find a similar depathological approach in the Hearing Voices Network, a peer support network that adopts a radical approach to the experience of hearing voices, seeing visions, or having other 'unusual perceptions' that others do not. First coming to the UK via Manchester in 1988, the approach avoids framing these perceptions as pathological 'imbalances in brain chemistry', and emphasises that these experiences can be seen as meaningful responses to the world. A common Hearing Voices mantra is that, instead of asking 'what's wrong with you?', we should ask: 'what happened to you?'

While the medical approach often emphasises voices and visions as a symptom of disorder, a Hearing Voices approach – which is practised at peer-led Hearing Voices support groups – might delve further into a person's perceptions, and how they respond to them. Are the voices saying something distressing, like telling you to harm yourself? What might happen if you spoke to them? Meanwhile, this non-pathologising approach makes space for the fact that some people find meaning or might even enjoy these experiences, for example accessing comfort, humour or friendship through the company of their voices. Some people say that their voices remind them of things they need to do, like packing a lunch or grabbing keys on the way to work. This process of reframing, accepting or analysing voices and visions can be deeply transformative; particularly if the fear of 'being Mad' exacerbates a person's distress. It can be all the more of a lifeline for people who have had damaging experiences with antipsychotic medication.

Jess Pons, who used to run Hearing Voices peer support groups, emphasises the importance of simply being with someone through their experience, without forcibly imposing any particular view of the world. She tells me:

If [a person] believes aliens exist, as someone walking alongside this person, I am humble and believe their reality. I may say I don't believe there are aliens trying to hurt us, but I am open to it, as who knows anything for certain? The dominant approach clings to certainty. Most humans cling to certainty to make sense of the world. To hold different explanations lightly, as I understand the Hearing Voices approach to do, does not sit well within the hierarchical clinical world of the dominant psychiatric approach.

The Hearing Voices approach is transformative because it rejects the idea of any singular 'objective reality', acknowledges that we all experience things differently, and what feels real varies from person to person. Almost all of us believe some things that most people do not, whether these beliefs are spiritual, political or otherwise. We all have the potential to see or hear things that are unusual or considered to 'not really be there' – when we think we hear someone say our name in a crowded room, or we look at an optical illusion. These things are not the same as the sometimes-frightening experiences that are categorised as psychosis. Rather, they are evidence of the fact that the difference between 'normal' and 'abnormal' perception is socially decided.

Depathologisation does not force us to embrace all elements of our disabilities as 'good', to stop taking medication, or to forgo all processes that currently fall under the umbrella of psychiatry and medicine. Rather, it is about rejecting zero-sum binaries of normal versus abnormal, healthy versus unhealthy, and embracing the messiness and nuance in between. It allows us to embrace an infinite spectrum of ways that we might relate to our bodyminds. These modes of relation can't be prescribed by any professional, and, like paint on a canvas, they can take any colour or shape that we want. Depathological approaches should, however, always be consensual, and should respect the different framings that people use to understand their material realities. Depathologisation represents another liberating possibility for thinking about distress, rather than a new dogmatic ideology to be universally enforced.

Beyond 'mental healthcare'

The projects described above are by no means exhaustive – and they can never be, because the ways that we think about and respond to our own minds are so personal, contextual, and varied. There is no one approach to trump them all. Some are in conflict with one another. But our minds are complicated, conflicting and ever-changing, and so our responses to mental health and Madness will need to be just as complex, multifaceted and dynamic too. A liberated future, for mental health, will always be nuanced, contradictory, plural and relentlessly tailored to each and every individual. As the prison abolitionist Mariame Kaba says: we need a million experiments.[6] There should be no paradigm or language that everyone has to adopt, no blanket response that can be applied to everyone.

This extends to how we think about treatment. We must hold the fact that one person's poison might be another person's tonic – that 'the answer' is not simply medication, psychoanalysis or meditation alone. 'Treatment' is usually understood through the narrow lens of Western medicine, but people find

6   https://millionexperiments.com/ (last accessed January 2023).

treatment in all kinds of places: in art, in talking, in intergenerational healing, in solidarity and community, in nature, in drugs, in moving their bodies, in particular physical spaces. Lots of people find joy and healing in activism, by coming together with others to remedy their material conditions. Most of us benefit from some combination of these things. We must reject the capitalist and austerity mindset[7] that demands a monolithic and limited approach to mental healthcare – it is whatever we want it to be. It will never be done, and it must increasingly expand beyond the things we even think of as 'mental healthcare'. Healing justice, for example, is a large-scale movement that attempts to intervene in cycles of intergenerational trauma and violence – simultaneously honouring indigenous knowledge and wisdom. This is a necessarily collective process. Care also means revolutionising not only our structures and systems, but revolutionising the ways that we relate to one another. Suffering is often relational – frequently stemming from conflict, abuse, or a lack of accountability. These modes of relation will also need to be transformed.

Our thinking has to be transformed too. Uncomfortable as it may be, there will never be 'an answer'. We must be agile, open to failure and criticism, able to scrap failed attempts and collect the fragments that worked, to respond to emotions as they change, and to the world as it changes too. This involves an embrace of *not knowing*,[8] of making space and humility to be wrong. Ultimately, it is only ever a good thing that our responses remain an unfinished sketch – not a final result, but a process.[9] We should keep sketching and erasing, dreaming and changing, towards a liberated future.

---

7   https://mentalhellth.xyz/p/disability-justice-and-mental-health (last accessed January 2023).

8   L. Ben-Moshe, 'Dis-Epistemologies of abolition', *Critical Criminology*, 26:3, (2018) pp. 341–55.

9   Ibid.

Conclusion

A future for mental health

When is the end of mental health? – Florence Oulds

This chapter contains a mention of suicide.

What is the future of mental health? Discussions around Madness/Mental Illness in the years to come constantly appeal to its complete obliteration: our own personal recoveries, the discovery of a gene, a medication, a miracle technology that brings an end to mental deviance. As Alison Kafer writes, illness and disability are seen as the sign of 'no future, or at least no good future'.[1] We often hear these ideas subtly reiterated on the left; for example, the idea that Madness/Mental Illness will cease to exist after capitalism. But these experiences have always existed, and will always continue to exist.

When it comes to suffering, in particular, we must invite this explicit contradiction into our vision for the future of mental health. While we should create the conditions for a world that produces less distress en masse, we must also transform the way that we think about distress itself; not only an unwelcome presence[2] to be forcibly controlled and eradicated. Suffering has always existed, whether it is those types designated as 'Madness/

---

1   Kafer, *Feminist, Queer, Crip.*
2   M. Shildrick, *Dangerous Discourse of Disability, Subjectivity and Sexuality* (New York: Palgrave Macmillan, 2009).

Mental Illness' or those that come in the form of grief, heart-break, long-term sadness or short-term fear. We should remove capitalist value judgments from our thinking about people's bodymind states, allowing them to make their own meanings and direct their own care and support. Our future must always provide space for Mad grief and Mad pride, for people who embrace their visions or voices, for people who claim their highest highs and their lowest lows even if we personally do not understand them. This cannot happen for Madness/Mental Illness alone – it must always be situated in our broader commitment to disability justice.

Throughout this book, I have built on the work of others to outline alternative directions for mental health support and care, acknowledging that I do not have all the answers. Into the twenty-first century, the state has continued to dismantle its mental health system. Many anti-psychiatry professionals of the 1960s would have supported this move. Anti-austerity leftists today, however, argue that we need to fund and expand mental healthcare. To avoid history repeating itself, we need to acknowledge in this climate that the reality is, paradoxically, both: of course we need more funding and resources, but we will not see revolutionary change if funding is pumped into carceral state structures that grew from the seeds of capitalism, not care. If abolition is about building 'life-affirming institutions', we need to invest in completely transformed approaches that sprout from different soil, divorced from the legacy of the capitalist asylum. We must champion alternative approaches that provide free, non-hierarchical, accessible, wide-ranging and community-controlled mental health support, to resist a right-wing neoliberal project of social murder through a combination of abandonment and control.[3] If we believe that

---

3   Spandler, 'From psychiatric abuse to psychiatric neglect?'

communities should have control over production, then it follows that we should have control over our healthcare and healing too. I have argued that this could look a million different ways, and that it is a necessarily messy project that requires that we imagine boldly while listening to everyone's needs. Crucially, it requires an end to the capitalist economic system, which has constructed our understanding of mental health and shaped the way that we approach it.

In a liberated future, care must take on new forms. All kinds of personalised care should be accessible to everyone, with near-infinite options to choose from: drugs, therapies, therapeutic communities – places to talk, places to create and places to stay with the freedom to leave. We should have the autonomy to blend and combine different types of care as we wish. There must be no coercion. No one can be kept in or kept out. We should embrace complexity in mechanisms that ensure the consent of all people, and prevent harm, even in the most difficult of situations. Impossibility, tension, contradiction and uncertainty will be things that we welcome and grapple with, rather than meet with fear and violent suppression. I hope that others will continue to build on these principles and craft more creative and specific responses to add to those I have detailed in the limited pages of this book.

All this can, of course, sit alongside our knowledge that Madness/Mental Illness is not a stable or coherent category at all. In any liberated future, we should see the end of 'illness' as a category that can be owned or controlled by any sort of state 'authorities', a bureaucratic rubber stamp that is our only possible ticket to care, and the difference between medicine or none, life or death. We all sit on the fringes of Madness/Mental Illness, so we should build a future where if you say you need help, you will be met with plenty. Support, healing and specialised knowledge should not be the property of the clinic or the GP's office, rather, it should be something that spills out onto the streets and into our homes. We have a lot to learn from the thinkers and activists who have long advocated for a 'radically socialised' approach to health, which acknowledges that having access to nourishing food, clean air and water, housing, light, art, creativity, connection, autonomy, support, and emotional fulfilment would do a greater deal for our wellbeing than the discovery of any new miracle drug or treatment. Social isolation, in particular, is one of the greatest 'risk factors' for suicide.[4] Why don't we start there?

The past and present of mental health has been dictated by capital, alienation, racism, colonialism, gendered oppression, psychiatric abuse, incarceration, gatekeeping and the enforcement of particular ways of knowing. The future must be something else. Although this project of liberation may never be finished, we should keep dreaming and imagining, out of our pain, into something that we can really live for.

---

4   L. Favril, R. Yu, A. Uyar, et al., 'Risk factors for suicide in adults: systematic review and meta-analysis of psychological autopsy studies', *Evidence-Based Mental Health*, 25, (2022), pp. 148–55.

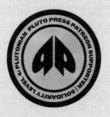

Thanks to our Patreon subscriber:

Ciaran Kane

Who has shown generosity and comradeship in support of our publishing.